From Here to Vitality

Processing the Psychological Side of Weight Loss

Carrie J. L. Hickman

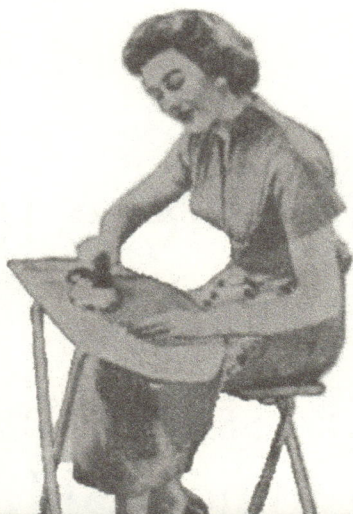

Permapress Publishing

Copyright © 2012 Permapress Publishing

Seattle, WA

All rights reserved.

ISBN-13: 978-0-9647949-0-0

DEDICATION

I want to express my heartfelt appreciation to and admiration for my dear wonderful husband, Steve. Steve, you are the light of my life, my soul mate, my best friend in all the world. Your support over these years has been invaluable. I'm so glad to be walking through life hand in hand with you! You are the BEST!

I have to share a little story, Dear Reader, that will give you a small taste of what my wonderful husband is like. I was fighting through an RA flare, sitting alone in our bedroom, sort of unconsciously singing as I was getting ready to write. He came into the room, his eyes red and swollen with tears he said, "I could hear you singing..." then of course seeing him I started to tear up... he continued, "It is the sweetest sound I have ever heard because I know when you sing you are feeling better." I am the luckiest person on the planet to be so loved.

SPECIAL THANKS

It takes a village to write a book. I want to thank my Mother for inspiring chapter one, and my son Joshua for inspiring the chapter on hard and soft rules and so much more. And I could never have gotten through this process without the love, support, encouragement, amazing ideas and editing skills of Micki Lechner-Riehle, Cheryl Scott Sweeney, and Robin Meyer. Micki you are the Gayle to my Oprah (or maybe it is the other way around). Cheryl you are my Soul Sista. And Robin you truly are my Hero. The three of you have been the most amazing friends anyone could hope for in this life! Your vitality inspires me!

CONTENTS

CARRIE J.L. HICKMAN

PREFACE

Everyone wants to know what diet is going to finally work for them! It's a lifelong quest for some of us. If this describes you, this book was designed to get you the answers you have wanted your whole life. I promise you that. Everyone knows that there is a psychological component to weight loss. We talk about it all the time, but only in the most vague terms. I am so excited to tell you that I stumbled upon a very old theory that when combined with the weight loss process makes it possible to process through the psychological side of weight loss and maintain your healthy weight for life! No more white knuckling it! No more hopping from one diet to another. No more unhealthy living! Imagine it! Every diet guru out there tells you that you must go through some kind of psychological processing, but they don't tell you how!

I was watching "The Biggest Loser" (I'm a huge fan. Even auditioned for the show once!) and I noticed that throughout each show, season after season they talk about the fact that there are psychological issues that we need to deal with in order to shed the weight and keep it off. This led me to look around a bit to see if any weight loss show or program had anything further to say on the subject. Turns out that they all know that many people with obesity have emotional issues to work through, but none of them seemed to know how to help us work through those issues. That's where this book comes in! That's the heart of this book. Working through this book will help you to address those issues and keep the weight off!! Dieting for the very last time! Finally getting past the issues that kept you overweight! That's exciting!

On the diet and exercise side, the very simply articulated program here is the difference between using someone else's diet plan, and knowing precisely what works for your body. It's evidence based science just for you! And you don't have to be a research scientist to get there!

Even though many stores may house this book in the diet section this is not exactly a diet book. It is, however, a diet companion book. It is about making changes in your life that will last a lifetime. Despite the fact that one chapter title is "What Should I Eat?" I will not tell you how or what to eat or what to do for exercise. I will however cover some basic realities about exercise, dieting, and about food just so that we are all on the same page. In addition, I will cover some of the best nutritional weapons we have against obesity. And although there are a lot of tips along the way, it isn't just a dieting tips book.

Who is Carrie Hickman? We are going to talk a lot about identity.

For now I will tell you that I am the mom of three amazing sons (and one little dog who imprinted on me like a duckling). I am the wife of a wonderful husband. We've been together now for over 24 years. I'm a sister, a daughter, an aunt, and a friend. And right now I am working on my doctorate in Research Psychology. I am not a personal trainer to the stars or a dietician. I have an MS in Psychology focused on researching health behaviors. I am honest, weak, inconsistent, tenacious, authentic, compulsive, and never ever air brushed. In other words, I am a lot like you.

Like many of you, I have this disease called obesity. In my life I have been thin and I have been heavy. Sometimes I am better able to manage my disease than at other times. Right now I am fighting a second disease which has made it really tough to fight obesity. Sounds like the perfect time to write this book, huh? <wry grin> I have RA. Like obesity, Rheumatoid Arthritis is a chronic, incurable disease. Because of this, I am not the muscle ripped model that the diet industry has trained you to dream of becoming. I have been close to that, but right now I am in the fight of my life against both obesity and RA.

This isn't a book just for people who are basically healthy who also happen to have obesity. It is also a book for those among us with other limitations like RA, fibromyalgia, diabetes, constant pain, etc. Most diet and exercise gurus focus on people who can exercise without restriction, whose abilities do not limit them. As a result their programs are not viable for the vast majority of us who have co-morbidities. A co-morbidity is the presence of one or more disorders (or diseases) in addition to a primary disease or disorder. Much more on that shortly. If you are basically healthy count your blessings! This will be much easier for you! If not, do not lose heart. This program was designed specifically to include you too.

I do want to caution you that when and if you decide to change your diet and begin to move more, you should consult your physician first. If you are seeing a psychologist or psychiatrist respect that relationship and talk with that person about your obesity. If you want, tell them about the book and ask them if they will participate in the process of your transformation. If they decide that this isn't a good time or program for you now, respect that. There is wisdom in that.

Take the information in this book, test it and make sure it works for you and that you are ready for this kind of radical change. Everyone knows there are emotional changes that must happen in order to lose weight and keep it off. But few people talk about how to make those changes and process through those emotions. There are eight steps in this program that will guide you through the psychological changes you need to make in order to keep the weight off permanently. This is your opportunity to create the life you have always wanted.

By the way, if you have a clinical diagnosis of obesity, buying this book can be tax deductible! You may not even know that you have this diagnosis, but if you have obesity, you know it. Ask your doctor if it is something in your record, and if not ask them enter it as a diagnosis. Then, anything you buy (including gym memberships) to deal with this disease is tax deductible as a medical expense! At least there's one advantage to having this disease!

DISEASE

I have to thank my mother who inspired me to begin with this important topic. I honestly thought that everyone understood that like any other chronic disease, obesity is incurable. But when you think about it, you know that many really smart people (even some doctors) think that weight loss is the cure for obesity. Weight loss is no more a complete solution for obesity than one insulin shot is a cure for diabetes. It is important that you understand why I say that obesity is a disease. In Feb. 2002 the Internal Revenue Service declared that obesity was, for tax purposes, a disease. This has allowed Americans to deduct expenses related to treating obesity on their taxes just the same way you would deduct any other medical expense. It is important that you have the diagnosis "obesity" from a doctor in order to get these benefits. Click on the words 'Internal Revenue Service' link above to read the law. The New York State Department of Health lists obesity as a chronic disease among others like diabetes, Arthritis, and Alzheimer's Disease and other Dementias. As early as 1997 an article in the Oxford Medical Journal, British Medical Bulletin declared, "Obesity is not a social stigma but an actual disease with a major genetic component to its etiology and a financial cost estimated at $69 billion for the USA alone" (Jung, 1997). I would make one small correction to that statement. I would say that Obesity is not JUST a social stigma....

More recently, Dr. Scott Kahan (2011) wrote a wonderful article on this topic that was published in the Huffington Post. Dr. Kahan went through the definition of a chronic disease and matched it point for point to obesity.

Following suit after Dr. Kahan, let's take a look at the definition of a chronic disease. A chronic disease is a disease that persists for a long time or is constantly recurring (Google Dictionary, 2012). Sounds like obesity to me. Disease simply means "dis-ease" in the body. That too sounds like obesity. When I am overweight I never feel at ease. More important though is how we define 'cure'. The way we are using the word (we aren't taking about smoking meats here) to cure is to restore to health; to relieve or rid of something detrimental, as an illness or a bad habit (Dictionary.com, 2012). That's appropriate for an approach to obesity. But to my knowledge, it isn't happening for most of us. 98% of dieters regain the weight they have lost within one year. That's not a cure. A chronic disease is chronic because there is no cure. Then by definition obesity is a chronic, incurable disease.

I'm hoping that is enough to convince you that if you have obesity, you have a chronic disease for which there is currently no cure. But if you are still wondering about this topic google it for yourself. There is a lot on this topic on the internet.

But an even bigger problem (if you can imagine) in the United States is our basic understanding of what constitutes an eating disorder. In this book I will be addressing the problems of people who live with an issue called disordered eating patterns; not eating disorders. How many Americans have disordered eating? This is a problem that affects approximately 5 million adults and their families in America alone (Hewitt et al., 2001). Many Americans have disordered eating and may not even know that they do and as a result the 5 million people mentioned above is probably just the tip of the iceberg! They aren't necessarily anorexic, super thin, or morbidly obese. They just eat compulsively or diet too much, exercise too much, or have some manner of eating that is chronically unhealthy for them. They may even eat a clean diet, but they smoke (or use some other addiction) to keep their compulsivity "in check". The compulsivity is still there; they are just exhibiting it in their other habits like smoking or over exercising. Any way you slice it they do not have a physically or psychologically healthy relationship with food or fitness. That's what an eating disorder is. The whole idea behind this book is to help you to develop a healthy, even curative relationship with food and to make peace with your body image. Become who you really want to be and be authentically healthy.

Further there is a lot of speculation that dieting may be an addiction in and of itself. The compulsive weighing and measuring of food (and of self for that matter) the constant fixation on food, the (short term) extreme vigilance, the rush you get when you first attempt a diet and the first few pounds come off, the crash cycle when it is over, could all be signs that dieting is an addiction. You must reflect on that, decide for yourself if that is an issue you need to attend to, and deal with it. If you are addicted to dieting, no diet will ever be your last. Food addictions can be addressed within this system, but the second book in this series will be focused completely on addictions and may offer more specific guidance in that regard.

I say all that to say that this book was not intended for use by people who have been diagnosed with eating disorders. This should in no way be a substitute for psychological therapy or a MD's involvement. Severe eating disorders are dangerous, and in all too many cases fatal, but they are not incurable. There is hope for people with eating disorders, but it takes time, work, and a lot of therapy. There are many people who have had severe eating disorders and through hard work on their behalf and on the part of their therapists, doctors, and families they got better. But this isn't that therapy. Help can be found at http://www.nationaleatingdisorders.org

In the same vein, this book is not a book about curing mental illness. Some psychological illnesses can contribute to obesity, no doubt about it. However, if you have trouble functioning due to psychological trauma or illness, please see a licensed clinical psychologist. A great resource for this is through the American Psychological Association. http://locator.apa.org

With all that we do know about the disease of obesity there is still a tremendous amount we do not know. For example, we don't know the cause of the disease. It is surely a combination of factors that include environment, genetics, and emotional health, but the brightest minds in the world still haven't sorted it out.

For now, you know that you have a disease that has no cure and for which the exact causes are still unknown. But that is not an indication that we are helpless in managing this disease. Quite the contrary, as with any chronic disease, you MUST MANAGE IT. And you must manage it every day for the rest of your life.

The problem is that there hasn't been a clear and effective way to help people do that. But with the help of science and psychology, you can manage it and in doing so you can live a healthy, vibrant life.

EVIDENCE

An evidenced-based healthy life is something most of us have never had the luxury, skills or focus to experience. It involves a highly personalized research-based diet and exercise program. Through this program you will be able to not only have the luxury of an evidenced based diet and exercise program, but be able to design and tweak this program as your needs change throughout your life. It is vital you understand the emotional underpinnings involved in keeping excess weight off. This program will address both the physical and the psychological aspects of weight loss and keeping it off.

Anyone can lose weight. Most of us have done it many times over. There is no mystery behind weight loss and no shortage of ways to do it. You need only to browse your local bookstore or online book retailer to get the enormity of this market. The only problem, and this is a big one... is that despite the claims of all these weight loss programs not one of them has mastered the art of keeping the weight off for a group larger than 2% of their membership. In fact, it is not in the diet industry's best interest to write books that show you how to keep the weight off for good. It would put them out of business!

So many diet gurus say, "this is not a diet, it is a lifestyle!" but they don't tell you how to create a lasting lifestyle. They may even say that you have to change how you look at things. But that's like saying, "You really should become a millionaire! If you really want it, you can do it!" But none of them tell you how to do that. You know it would take changing your life and examining your emotions around food, but they never tell you how to do that. That's because even the well meaning diet and exercise gurus don't know that in order to create lasting change you must create a new identity that supports that change. And even if they can tell you that you need to change your identity, they can't tell you how to create a new identity. Rest assured, this book does just that.

So you have tried them all, maybe even had weight loss surgery. Does that mean it is too late for you? Not in the least! In fact, that's my own story. I too have this incurable disease called obesity. I have fought with it most of my life, even had gastric bypass to try to cure it! Most of my efforts were successful for a short time. Even weight loss surgery was only successful for me for a few years. But I am grateful for those experiences because it was those experiences that led me to understand this issue in a way I could never have understood it from an outsider's (thin, healthy) perspective.

This book was borne from my PhD work in psychology. My dissertation was focused on people who had weight loss surgery and understanding how and why some kept the weight off, while others (a very large and growing number in fact) regained the weight. I was so inspired by the research that I had to do something concrete, something applied to help people who have searched the world over for the best diets and exercise for them. Most of us don't have a degree in nutrition or exercise physiology. Putting our own program together without the raw tools and education would be impossible if not foolhardy until now. I have already stated that I am not a nutritionist or a physical trainer. True. But I know about research and like you I can log and keep good records of what I do each day. That's all the science you need to know!

So what is an evidence-based diet program?

It is a completely and honestly individualized plan, based on the research data that you provide. The results you get provide the evidence of your program's success! You can log both physical and psychological data points as you go through your day (based on a variety of psychological questionnaires in the program). This isn't about using a calorie counter that's going to spit out simple facts like if you eat 1000 calories a day you will lose 2 pounds a week. That kind of thing is built on averages and for individuals is fairly meaningless. Using this program, you will be able to discover specifically how much you should eat of what kinds of foods that work naturally with your own body to produce higher levels of energy, more productivity, better moods, and of course lasting weight loss. No more national averages! You are not average. Why should you follow a statistical model built on the average?

And this is a program that you can update and tweak for the rest of your life. Your body and mind will change with age and as such it is vital to being able to go back to the program and reassess your energy levels, productivity, etc. It is important that when you see your energy flailing, you know why and how to fix it. If you find you have more aches and pains or depression, it is vital to know what kinds of things you must change in order to combat those changes in your body and your mind.

This isn't for the faint of heart. It takes determination that's for sure. But it doesn't involve taking pills, or buying pre-prepared foods, having surgery, or being addicted to anything. It does not involve trying to look like a celebrity model, or paying a personal trainer to yell at you. It especially doesn't involve some big corporation that has a patent on "the latest weight loss pill" making millions on your frustration. And it doesn't involve spending your life white-knuckling it, just to stay thin.

It does involve you getting to know who you are, where you've come from, where you are going, and how all that effects you and why you are overweight. That is a tall order for anyone.

I talk a lot throughout this book about writing, keeping logs, journaling, and making notes. If you hate to write, don't. There are tools now that can fairly accurately convert voice to text. Technology today means there is really no excuse for not taking a closer look at your life. Someone once told me many years ago that 'you learn as your write' and I have confirmed that many many times over since then. I believe that it is therapeutic and can yield remarkable results when we simply write things down. Of course, that is just the start of what we are doing together.

This book is all about becoming who you always wanted to be. It is about being the best you can be. It's about living an authentic, healthy life; the life where who you are on the inside shines out through vitality and health and energy. If you are up to that, hop aboard! You are about to take the ride of your life!

Take a minute to write a list of the areas you want to study about yourself. Diet and exercise are fundamental. Moods are vital. Habits and practices are areas you should be well aware of in order to understand what is contributing to your disease. Make a list of what healthy behaviors you have used in the past and then keep a record of when you engage in them over the next week or two. Now make a list of unhealthy behaviors, when and how you engage in them. Are you a smoker? When and where do you smoke? Over eating should be noted along with associated emotions, times, and places.

Start a log that you keep over the next month. As you read you will add more and more to it. Watch for patterns in emotions and eating habits as well as places and times that are triggers for unhealthy behaviors.

AUTHENTICITY

This is the goal. The goal of this book, and of (I believe) life itself, is to live an authentically integrated healthy life. I use that expression a lot, so I think it is prudent to look at exactly what I mean by that. The goal is not to be "skinny" or to look like a model. The goal isn't even just weight loss for the sake of losing weight. The goal is much bigger, deeper, and more important than that. Whether or not you realize it, your life is integrated. Your moods, your energy levels, your sense of purpose, your weight, eating habits, exercise practices, health problems and illness, your values, your productivity and more, are all integrated and reflect your vitality. Vitality is simply your potential for life.

When we choose a weight loss program, for example, we are facing an avalanche of options. Every single one of those options is represented by a spokesperson or a model (maybe several models some of whom look like 'ordinary people') who have supposedly used that weight loss program to lose weight. Some of them have. But buyer beware! What you don't know is far more important than what you know about these cases.

All you know about those models or spokespeople is that they say that they have used a certain method to lose weight and for them it worked. What you do not know is... well anything else about them and their health status. Generally you don't know how healthy their mind is in relationship to food. What you are seeing is no more than a snap shot. One single frame in time of a person's life. In that frame everything looks amazing. The person looks happy, healthy, and successful. Do you really know that they are? It is the job of the marketing department to make those models look as good and as happy and as healthy as they can possibly look, so that you will want to look like them!

Here's the reality. Even if you lost weight, you would likely not look like a model. You will still be you. You have no idea if that model even uses the program they say they do, and if they have used it, how long and how closely they have followed it. You have no idea if that model is clinically depressed, how productive his or her life is, or if they are indeed healthy at all. You don't know if that model is throwing up 5 times a day because she can't stop eating, but is desperate to keep her weight off. You don't know if the photos of the models are genuine or if they have been air brushed. There is a literal mountain of information that you do not know about the program, the models, the long term effects of any particular diet. What we do know is that many programs are simply unhealthy and packed with lies designed to make money. They are untrustworthy.

I was a model like that, in a small sense. After my gastric bypass and the subsequent weight loss, I was asked to speak at several events about my experience. I can tell you that in that snapshot of my life, I was thin and that made me happy. And it was great, as long as I had no hunger sensation. That lasted about two years. When my hunger sensation returned I could no longer eat 500 -700 calories a day without feeling starved and food obsessed. I could not run enough each day to keep up with the calorie burns, and naturally I began to put on weight. When I was struck with RA, the problem compounded itself because I could no longer run (or exercise the way that I had). Compound that with RA drugs that encourage weight gain and there was literally no hope for me to keep the weight off.

More important than all of that, I knew that the results I had through gastric bypass were temporary for me. I had not dealt with my propensity to use food as an emotional coping mechanism. I had not changed myself in any way emotionally. I was not whole and I felt like my success was not authentic. By that I mean that I had not worked through the hard stuff (emotional pain, etc.) I knew was still inside me. On the outside I looked successful, but inside I was still the fat person I had always been, still crying for help.

What is Success?

We have been conditioned through the media, and yes even through the medical and governmental establishment, to measure successful fitness and weight loss by the numbers. Specifically we have been trained to watch our weight and or body mass index. While it is clear why these kinds of objective measurements were chosen, they have begun to lose meaning.

The government and medical establishment had to have an "objective measure" that most people could easily understand, when communicating health issues. This is how certain weight and BMI and even blood pressure and cholesterol numbers came to be understood as either healthy or unhealthy. However, as time has gone by the medical community has changed what the numbers mean. The numbers that indicate that a person is a healthy weight have changed over the decades. Recommendations for healthy blood pressure numbers have recently changed too. As doctors find out more about what constitutes health, these numbers and their meanings will continue to change.

Being a specific weight isn't something that our government can simply hand to us. One size does not fit all! The weight charts are based on statistics. You need to know what weight you are most comfortable and healthy living at. For example, when I had lost 100 pounds after gastric bypass I was really thin for my frame. Unfortunately, the BMI recommendations still said that at 140 pounds I was overweight. I'm 5'3" and in order to satisfy the "BMI gods" I would have to be more like 120 pounds to be considered a "healthy weight". So, I allowed myself to continue to lose weight until I was at about 125 pounds. Trouble was at that weight I was constantly blacking out and even passed out twice! And it was clear to everyone who knew me that I was way too thin at that weight. You must have a scientifically based way to know what weight is healthiest for you. We will get there, I promise you.

Living an authentically healthy life means simply that your mind and body are in sync. It means that you live an integrated, holistic life. I like the connection between the words integrated and integrity. Both words revolve around the concept of being whole. Success is more about living a comfortable, energetic, productive long life than living life at a certain weight. By that I mean that success has more to do with not being sick and tired than what your BMI can tell you. We are moving toward vibrancy and energy and away from sickness and early unnecessary death.

BMI is highly regarded as one of the most accurate current measurements for health, but it should not be. BMI was never meant to be used in this way, nor does it accurately measure health. BMI is a formula devised by an astronomer in the 1830s that measures height and weight and nearly a century later we are attempting to use it to create a "statistical norm" that could be used as an objective measure for health. The biggest problem with BMI is that it doesn't differentiate between fat and muscle. Muscle weighs more than fat, and as a result you can be a very fit body builder with a terribly unhealthy looking BMI. That is not the case for most people who have obesity. But it is a major failing of the BMI measure.

The point here is that weight and BMI can tell us some things, but are in no way the whole story. Nor should they be the sole measure of health.

An authentically healthy life is one that is focused on bringing what we know about being healthy into our experience. The idea is to behave in a way that is consistent with our understanding of what constitutes a healthy life. The first problem is to truly understand what it means to be healthy. The second part is to them choose to live according to what we understand.

Health encompasses a vast amount of things more than just height and weight. Health is mood, it is clarity of thought, it is productivity, it is energy, and it is having your own purpose in life. In short, it is about vitality. Vitality encompasses all those things we can measure about our health. Your vitality score should reveal your energy levels, moods, pain levels, and productivity, weight, sense of purpose, and disease progression. If you are vital and fully alive, you vitality scores will be higher. If any part of your health is flagging, you vitality scores will reflect that in a lower score.

When we do not behave in accordance with our beliefs about what would make us healthy, we cause something called cognitive dissonance. Cognitive Dissonance is the state of having inconsistent thoughts, beliefs, or attitudes, especially as related to behavioral decisions and attitude change (google dictionary, 2012). Cognitive dissonance makes us uncomfortable, and in some cases, miserable. We know that liquid diets will cause weight loss, yet when we choose a liquid diet we can have a great amount of cognitive dissonance about whether it is healthy for us. Most of us understand that these diets only work temporarily at best, so all through the struggle of using this kind of plan we know that eventually we will go back to eating solid food and that it likely means our weight loss will vanish and all our hard work and suffering will be for nothing.

At what weight are you most energetic? The height and weight charts and BMI calculators do not take energy into account. If you are passing out because being 118 pounds is too small for your metabolism, it is not a healthy weight for you. This despite what the weight charts say.

We want to know before we choose a diet plan that it works, and that it is likely to work for us. The media short cut for this is to create a model with the image that will reassure us that if it worked for her, it can work for us. They will tell us that in pretty much those exact words! "If it worked for me, it can work for you!" They do not know you. They cannot possibly know that it will work for you. Maybe the diet is a liquid diet packed with sugar and maybe you have diabetes! That won't work for you! But they don't know that because despite what their ad says, they do not know you.

Then the next step the diet industry takes is to choose someone admired from Hollywood, or some amiable public face, and make them their spokesperson. Just because you like someone, does not mean that you are like them. It doesn't mean that your health journey can be just like theirs. It doesn't actually mean anything except that you enjoy, respect, or have positive thoughts about the spokesperson. It is the goal of marketing to associate the diet with the spokesperson to bring a more likability to the product. I like Jessica Simpson, but that doesn't mean I like weight watchers or think it is the best I can do for my body. Frankly, I don't know Jessica Simpson. But the Weight Watchers folks sure hope that because I like Jessica Simpson some of my admiration for her will rub off on their diet program! They hope that the credibility of doctors will rub off onto their programs. They hope that if they show us someone who is beautiful, we will associate beauty with their diet plan. It's marketing 101. Credibility by association.

And if a diet or exercise commercial carries the disclaimer that reads something like, "results are not typical" you should take that to heart. Why do we see that disclaimer, and then think we will be the exception to the rule? It's not because our self confidence is so high that we just know we can do it, against the odds. It is because while they are running that disclaimer that means most people are not successful with their programs, they are contradicting it verbally. They are telling us that we CAN do it. That this is the one diet plan that WILL FINALLY WORK for us. And while that little tiny printed disclaimer at the bottom of the screen is saying it won't work for most people, (98% in fact) the more powerful message is the one we hear. And this is by design. This is how our brains work!

While we might read the disclaimer once, the spokes model keeps repeating the contrary message over and over and over again. This way, we are getting the verbal message many times while we might not even read the tiny written disclaimer once. The diet guru wants us to get the message that we can do it, not the message they must tell us by law, that most people cannot do it. Make no mistake, if it wasn't required by law, it would not be there at all.

So, if the results they are showing are not typical, what are the typical results??

Typically, these products and diet plans do not work.

TYPICALLY.

That means that for 98% (that is a research statistic, by the way) of the folks who try their darnedest to succeed, spend their money, and work like crazy, will regain any weight they lose within one year. It is a hard fact, but in this sense, you are typical.

Authenticity is the key. Are all the aspects of your life that effect your health consistent with one another? Are your mood, energy, productivity, clarity of thought, reflected in your diet and weight? What do mood, energy, productivity and clarity of thought, sense of purpose, have to do with how much you weigh? If you suffer from obesity, maybe everything.

REALITIES

There are a whole lot of problems that can and usually do accompany obesity. It is a disease like a lot of others, which has a range of symptoms and causes. As you begin to approach managing this disease there are some realities with which you should be familiar. Obesity is a very complicated disease. If not, medical scientists and psychologists would have cured it by now. Given that reality, we have to approach obesity with a few other realities in mind. The first reality is that you are in for the fight of your life. You are literally fighting for your life. No metaphor intended at all. Obesity kills. The problems that obesity causes for your heart, lungs, and veins can take your life. This isn't a vanity thing. The hard cold reality is that obesity is deadly and you must manage it before it kills you. Left untreated, this disease is deadly. Treating it ineffectively can make the disease a lot worse over time.

Reality number two: Obesity is painful, both physically and emotionally. That fact alone makes it difficult to fight. Exercise is painful when you have obesity. Even walking can be painful. But movement is REQUIRED for life. You cannot be a healthy person if you do not move. Even if you are disabled, movement is still required for life. Further, since you have the disease of obesity, your requirements for movement are MORE than if you did not have this terrible disease. Does that seem unfair? Sure, it's unfair. Is it unfair when a child gets cancer? Of course! All diseases are an unfair part of life. Does that mean that you get to sit around eating spaghetti off a plate on your chest watching "The Biggest Loser" because life has been unfair to you? Nope. Is it unfair that we who suffer from obesity can't eat the same way that our naturally thin best friend can? Yup. The whole thing is unfair. That's the third reality.

The fourth reality is that keeping the weight off requires work. For the rest of your life you will work. Once you finish this program the work will be a lot easier, but it will take management. Many of us (me included) are not great at the day to day management of anything. We have automated our car and house payments, and just about everything else we can. But this is not something you can automate. You can NEVER ever again rest on your laurels. You can never ever again think that once you lose the weight that your obesity is cured forever. It is one of the fundamental realities of our

13

lives. You must spend time EVERY SINGLE DAY doing good things for your body, both in terms of diet and in terms of exercise, regardless of how you feel. Further, you must manage your moods, productivity, and general vitality as a part of managing your weight or you will fail.

The diet part is easy. If you follow the one rule I have for what to eat you will never have a problem with food. Just remember to ask yourself if what you are about to eat is the best, most nutritious food you can eat. If it is, eat it. If not, make another choice. You live in a society so privileged that you get to choose the best thing for yourself every time you eat. See chapter 8 for details.

Many people who suffer from obesity (and I mean literal suffering) have a difficult time exercising. The biggest problem is that exercise hurts when you have obesity. Heck, it can hurt when you are fit! But when you have obesity, consistent exercise becomes complicated. And notice that I said consistent exercise. The problem is for folks who want to exercise but have a physical limitation like obesity, exercise, especially at first, can complicate your physical limitations. Let me explain.

When you first begin an exercise program it will take 2-3 weeks before you get past being sore and miserable. That's if you are basically healthy. If you have obesity and other co-morbidities like I do, that window of stiffness and soreness can be much longer and much more intense. (more about co-morbidities here)

One of the common problems for many people with obesity is that we tend to be compulsive about everything in our lives. That includes food and that also includes exercise. While we can turn that compulsivity into a positive for ourselves, the beginning of any program is not the time to be compulsive. The philosophy of "if a little is good, more is better" will not work for you at the start of most programs. You know what I am saying. You've been here before. Many many times, some of you. You get all revved up and decide that you are going to get the weight off so you go on a starvation diet eating only green olives and black coffee and you work out for 3 hours a day after which time you sit in an ice cold bathtub to burn calories. You also know that it takes about 3 days before you can no longer maintain that and you quit; defeated, crushed and your self-esteem in tatters.

A note about self-esteem. Self-esteem is only built when you accomplish something. It isn't built on how many times you are complimented, or how skinny you look in your jeans. It isn't even built on positive self talk in the mirror every day, or some fitness guru yelling his mantra at you. Self-esteem can only be earned by working hard toward a goal and reaching that goal. If you have never worked hard to reach a goal your self-esteem is probably not as healthy as it could be. For some reason in our culture we think that our self-esteem is low because we haven't been told we are good looking. It has nothing to do with that at all!

The important thing about building self-esteem is that the more difficult the goal, the longer it takes to achieve, and the more you put into reaching that goal, the more you will get out of it in terms of lasting, positive self-esteem. Working toward a PhD is difficult and it takes a relatively long time. It is a worthwhile thing to do that is good for my self-esteem. Losing weight and keeping it off is very very difficult and takes a lifetime of management. That translates into something that will do a whole lot for your self-esteem. And it is the gift that keeps on giving. As each anniversary passes, each healthy year you mark on the calendar can represent an amazingly difficult goal achieved. This goal is so difficult that scientists and personal trainers and weight loss specialists the world over haven't cracked it. But you can. You can. This is your new reality.

Reality number five is that the next time you complain to yourself or someone else that your self esteem is low, what you are saying is that you haven't really tried hard or pushed yourself to accomplish enough worthy goals. It's not about getting support from someone else. It's about pushing yourself past your known limits. Pushing past where you are comfortable, and truly accomplishing something important.

Some of us have accomplished important things, but fail to recognize them. That's a different problem, and I think it is rare for Americans. But the bottom line is, when you set out to achieve a goal, create a situation in which you will be successful. Then celebrate those successes. They aren't bragging points. They are your self esteem. Self esteem literally means "how you see yourself". It is important you see yourself with pride in your accomplishments.

Reality number six is that if you have co-morbidities or what I call "Complex obesity" you are going to have more difficulty treating and managing your disease than those who suffer "simple obesity". Complex obesity comes from having co-morbidities (click the bold words above for definitions). These co-morbidities can be caused by obesity or can cause obesity. This is something that is different for each person.

Again, this isn't fair. Not much about life is fair.

If you understand RA you will understand why I make this point. It is not an excuse, but part of my reality. The medicines I must take to keep Rheumatoid Arthritis at bay also cause weight gain. Exercise is nearly impossible, despite the fact that just 4 years ago I was a long distance runner and I love exercise. I'm not some Barbie Doll with six pack abs and the ability to do back flips. I'm here in the trenches with you. And I am here for life. Just like you.

I am determined, despite my illness to be as healthy as possible in both body and mind. I am determined to be authentically healthy. I say all this to encourage you. Our lives are complicated. We all have roadblocks, pain, lack of motivation, maybe depression, and many of us have illnesses that constantly contribute to our weight gain or regain. These are our realities.

But if I can do this I believe that nearly anyone can. If constant intractable pain and medicines that cause weight gain can't stop me, there is hope for you too. Keep in mind, that's not the same as saying, "it worked for me, it can work for you too!" The difference is the context. We are specifically talking here about potential excuses in this context, not in general terms about an unknown diet plan. Co-morbidities are excuses in empathetic disguises some have called 'reasons'. Your own plan has to be based on evidence generated completely by you, for you.

Another reality that simply must be addressed is imperfection. We all know we are not perfect, we never can be. Positive self esteem has nothing to do with being perfect. It is our reality that we live in an imperfect world. Therefore, no matter how well meaning you are you (like me) will slip into old patterns from time to time. I just slipped this week! I had some blood sugar issues due to my gastric bypass and I panicked. The panic made me temporarily lose focus just long enough to eat red meat, specifically a hamburger. It was available, and I had reverted. That was all it took to jolt me back into reality. Within 12 hours the joints in my hands were swollen and painful, my back pain had returned, and I was constipated. All signs of inflammation. The point isn't that I slipped back into old patterns. The point is that when I did I saw the results and stopped myself before the old pattern could reinstate itself as a practice. I told you, I am a lot like you. I know you slip. No worries, your secret is safe with me! <wink> But don't let the inevitable guilt turn one slip into a practice. And don't let it rob you of your accomplishments so far.

I'd love to tell you that after 9 months without red meat my appetite for it has completely disappeared. Life would be so much easier that way! But I can't tell you that. And I can't tell you that birthday cake isn't tempting. What I can tell you is that if you have just one small piece, if won't kill you. You might be miserable afterward, maybe enough to make you regret eating it. But it won't kill you.

The reality adjacent to this one is that food has few negative short term consequences for most of us. This might sound positive on first blush, but it isn't. The fact is that we think enough about the long term. The problems that food causes us are generally long term, and because of our shortsightedness, it is easy to forget about the long term problems food causes.

In a way, I'm lucky. RA has "gifted" me with the ability to see the immediate effects of inflammation in my body in a way most folks don't often see. And gastric bypass surgery has lowered my tolerance for sugar and fat. You might be like my friend Rosie whose inflammation shows up in her intestines. But for many of us the negative short term consequences just aren't apparent.

It's a lot like smoking. I've never been a smoker, so my information is strictly second hand. (Unless you count pretending to smoke when I was 12 sitting on a trail with my friends in the woods near my childhood home.) From what I gather, the immediate effects of smoking are generally positive. It's calming and is a stimulant, similar to caffeine. I get that. I'm a coffee drinker. It acts on receptors in the brain to make you feel good. But we all know the long term side effects of smoking, and for some of us that is enough of a deterrent. I'm more afraid of lung cancer than any positive short term affect a cigarette could have. Sadly, it is possible to have the same fear and be completely addicted to smoking, unable to stop. That, my friend is a hellish way to live. If you are there, you have my sympathy. (Watch for the next book in this series. I'm planning a book focused on addictions.)

The problem with food is that unlike addictions, you obviously can't simply quit it. There's no way I know of to live a healthy life without food. We must learn to cope with our addictive, compulsive, and unbalanced relationship with food (and other unhealthy substances and activities that we practice). There is no way around it. Many diet and fitness gurus will tell you that you do not need to change your lifestyle. BS. Unless you come into alignment with who you want to be, you will never do anything in life but struggle with your relationship to food.

One way that I cope with the compulsive tendencies within myself is to choose healthy things to eat compulsively. For example, celery or ice chips. Ice cubes may hurt your teeth, but smaller ice chips are pretty benign. I did break a tooth on ice cubes once, so be aware there are some risks with those. The idea is that if I feel the need to eat something, but I am not truly hungry, eating one of these two things generally saves me from myself. You may find something quite different that will help you curb your compulsive behaviors. I know people who brush their teeth when they feel like this. That did not work for me. Others go for a walk. Some people automatically want to eat when they watch TV. I know one person who replaced her sofa with a treadmill and she walks while watching and doesn't let herself watch anything without walking. Chewing ice works for me because I can count it toward my daily water intake and it is calorie free. Besides, I like it.

Living a life of vitality doesn't happen by accident. It's not "natural" for those of us with obesity. It does not happen automatically. This was a big realization for me. I hope you are hearing that you must live a deliberate life in order to live with vitality and health. That's just reality.

Write Your Story

Make a list of your realities. What health issues do you face?

What social issues make it difficult for you to be healthy?

How will you deal with these realities in the coming months?

Make a plan to work around them, with them, and to overcome some of them.

SOFT RULES & HARD RULES

Whether we are aware of them or not, we all employ soft rules and hard rules in our lives. For example, it is a hard rule in my life that I do not smoke cigarettes. I never smoke cigarettes and plan to continue in this practice throughout my life. The problem is not with following hard rules, those are easy. It's the soft rules you've got to watch out for. Soft rules are those quasi-rules that we set up for ourselves which may or may not be important. The big distinction between hard and soft rules is that breaking them has no immediate consequence. Soft laws are guidelines. It's like a behavior wish list. Because soft rules are just guidelines they are very easily broken. After all, the consequences are not painful when we break our own soft rules.

The big problem for people who suffer with obesity is that diet is often a collection of soft rules. We use soft rules to guide our dietary intake, rather than hard rules primarily because it seems easier. It allows for us to "cheat" and allows for variances that would otherwise not be allowed. Cheating on a diet is an absurd concept. It amounts to cheating on yourself. Why would you do that? It is short term thinking and the result of a lack of self respect. It has to do with a momentary pleasure that wrecks havoc on your body and your metabolism for what could be a long time. It's not even self centeredness. If you are truly self centered you would have your own best interests at heart. But cheating on yourself is just childish. Grow up. Think long term. Ask yourself if what you are doing can be sustained until you are 90 or 100 years old. If not, don't do it.

I just heard a story about a man in his 30s who for the past 9 or 10 years has refused sugar, including a small slice of his own birthday cake. At first blush it sounds extreme, and completely unbalanced. But what if you learned that same man has had type two diabetes for the past 9 or 10 years? That changes everything. Suddenly what looked out of balance seems perfectly respectable and honorable! People who have type two diabetes must for the sake of their health, restrain from eating large amounts of sugar.

In the same way, if you suffer from obesity you must have some hard rules that might at first seem extreme to someone who does not suffer obesity. You must continually and faithfully fight this disease or it will inevitably kill you.

Take heart dear Ones. Hard rules are easier to follow than soft rules. Once you have decided to make something a hard rule, it is much easier to follow through with than if you think of it as a simple guideline.

So, what hard rules must you employ in your life to be healthy? I'm not saying that everything in life must be rigid, but there are things you must do to manage your disease. Unmanaged obesity simply contributes to ill health. Want to feel better? Live more? Take your diagnosis seriously and treat the disease!

Hard rules that everyone should look at incorporating into their lives include movement. For a detailed look at movement, check into chapter 10. Even if you are a paraplegic, this applies to you. If you are ambulatory, you must move every single day of your life. A good rule is to give yourself one day a week when your movement is lighter than the other six days. Here's why this is important.

Moving six days a week and taking one day a week off is a slippery slope for many people. Moving every single day is a no-brainer. You know that if you wake up in the morning you have a duty to yourself to move in a therapeutic way. The baseline is to drip sweat for 30 minutes a day. Chapter ten has more detail on this. Every single day of your life if you are a diabetic, you must measure your blood sugar and take the appropriate amount of insulin. You don't wake up one day and decide that today you're going to take an insulin holiday. That would be ridiculous, and dangerous. In the same way if you have a thyroid disorder you can't just treat it six out of seven days a week. You must take your medicine every single day.

I know a lot of personal trainers support the notion of one day off physical training per week. It is important if you are training hard that your body has some time to recover. I do not disagree with that. However, I would say that since we are not (in all likelihood) training for a professional sporting event, you can still allow your body to recover by making one day a week a less intense day.

This has another advantage over the one day a week off method. When you exercise it changes your brain chemistry. Working out for six days and then stopping altogether for one day can have a debilitating effect on your moods. It may not happen on your day off, but it might. It is more likely to happen on the day that follows your day off. Depression and negative emotions like anger and sadness can wash over you like a flood when your work out schedule is interrupted suddenly. This can cascade into a lack of motivation to move which can further your depression and negative emotions. Your whole program can derail in a matter of days.

Further, the rule that you have created that says you "need" a day off from exercise can morph into a point of convenience for events that come up. You are attending a wedding and rather than getting up early to exercise you count the wedding day as your day off. Wedding celebrations can leave one with a hangover, which shoots the next day's movement too! Then your normal day off comes around and it is easy to take that day off too. It's easy from there to begin to see your exercise as a soft rule that has no real dire consequences. After all, that week went by and you might not have gained any weight at all. That is only because the consequences of not moving daily are long term and for the most part cannot be seen in the immediate short term.

I want to caution you in terms of your "less intense day" and what you choose to do. If you are a walker or jogger on six days of the week, make your less intense day something that you consistently do. For example, swim on those days. Play a game outside with your family that day. Take a stroll with your sweetheart, or your grandma. Join a baseball league that has practice one day a week. Whatever you do, be consistent with it. It is as important as the six other days. It is important that you make it a hard rule and as much a priority as the other six days. It is all too easy to let the concept of a less intense day become less than it should be. "I've played outside for 10 minutes. That's movement, right?" If you do not make this a hard rule, before you know it you will be getting into the one day off trap.

Another area people have a difficult time with is drinking enough water. It is vital to your therapy against obesity that you drink enough water to allow your body to flush the fat out. Without it you will not lose weight. Later we will address the water issue in detail. For now it is important that you make drinking water a hard rule.

What do I mean when I say "water"? I mean water. I mean clean tap water. If you live in an area where your tap water isn't clean you might have to purify it in some way. For the vast majority of us, the water that is pumped into our homes is clean and sufficient. Unless you live in a developing nation, you probably do not have to worry about this issue.

I am not talking about sweetened drinks, coffee, or tea. Herbal tea that contains no caffeine or sweetener is okay. But adding artificial sweeteners, sugar, or honey is not. Water, like everything else is an acquired taste. After you have 'forced' yourself to drink your 8- 8oz glasses a day, plus another 8 oz. glass for every 10 pounds you are overweight, you will find your natural thirst returning to you. I remember thinking, 'I just drank a ton of water, why am I so darned thirsty?' Because you body likes it, and will continue to ask for more. That makes it easy to keep it up. Pure clean water is important to every organ, your skin, intestines, blood pressure; your whole body benefits from water. Best of all it is highly therapeutic in the fight against obesity.

A well hydrated body allows you to lose fat. It is that simple. A dehydrated body will tend to hold onto fat. By dehydrated I don't mean that you've gone for days without water and you are dragging yourself across the desert. Many of us are dehydrated and do not know it. We eat when we are thirsty, rather than drinking. We drink too many caffeine laden drinks and sweetened drinks that do not allow us to process fat and toxins. If you understand that the only way to lose fat from your body is through urine or sweat, you understand how therapeutic it is to be well hydrated. The more water you drink, the more you pee and sweat and that leads to the right kind of weight loss; fat.

Here's a biggie! Eat only for nutrition. Wow. Make that a hard rule and you have the key to health in your hand. If you make it a hard rule for yourself that when you are emotionally upset you do not allow yourself to eat, you will save yourself a tremendous amount of calories and long term heartache. The issue is this: you must have a readily available means for coping with your stress.

Plan ahead. Hard times will come. Create a coping mechanism for yourself that you can easily grab when you are in a difficult emotional situation. The problem is that it is difficult, nearly impossible, to replace food as a coping mechanism if you do not plan ahead. Simply having something available that will help you cope, isn't enough. You must spend time doing the activity that will help you cope when you are not involved in an emergent or emotional situation. If you simply grab a stress ball and declare that you will use it instead of eating to cope with stress you are likely to fail. If the stress ball isn't therapeutic for you, it isn't going to help you. You must practice using it.

I'm not advocating or disparaging stress balls, it is a simple example. Many people will need a much more elaborate plan to cope with stress than that. Whatever you chose, practice calming yourself at the end of the day using your new tool. I find a hot cup of tea and a mystery book at the end of the day calm me down from the normal stressors of each day. I usually read myself to sleep at night. It is a form of practice for me.

For some people smoking cigarettes is something they do when they are out at a bar socializing and drinking. I would challenge you to rethink these kinds of practices. Not because one cigarette every month or so will give you lung cancer, but because you are in effect practicing an unhealthy behavior that makes you feel good. Why is that important? It's important because the things you practice that make you feel good are things that can very soon become the coping mechanisms you reach for in dark times.

As a gastric bypass patient I have had to adopt a rule concerning eating very slowly. It is a good rule in general, but essential for folks who have had gastric bypass. What it means is that for every meal I eat with others I am the last one eating when everyone else is finished (and generally gone from the table, or wish they could be). But it also means that generally speaking, food doesn't get 'stuck'. That's important because when food gets stuck it causes me severe pain. And even though it was a rule for me for years it took an understanding of hard and soft rules in order to really commit to it. Now I have made it a hard rule.

The great thing about hard rules is that the longer you practice them, the stronger you become with regard to that behavior. Smoking for example, holds no Temptation for me what-so-ever. I determined as a teenager after sneaking around and trying it a handful of times, that I would never do it again. And I never have. Similarly, it is a hard rule for me that I will never cheat on my husband. After 24 years of faithful marriage it has no hold on me at all. I have no desire to do anything even close to that. I have made it a practice not to think about it or allow it to consume me in any way. In this way I was drawn farther and farther from it as each year passed. I am sure there are areas in your life where you have employed hard rules that you simply live by now. They have become a part of your identity.

That's the whole point of this program. You must incorporate your priorities into your identity in order to make them permanent in your life. Is your health a priority? Incorporate healthy behavior into your identity. Practice healthy behaviors.

The more difficult part about hard rules is that they can drift into soft rule territory very easily if we are not mindful. For example, I know that eating wheat is problematic for me. For a long time I would begin by not eating bread which is the most obvious thing in our culture that contains wheat. But eating meat or fish that is breaded, particularly on a road trip seems to be a particular weakness for me. I think I am doing ok by ordering a salad with meat, even when the meat is breaded. After a short time of allowing that compromise I am more likely to compromise even more and eat just certain kinds of bread like sourdough, or sprouted grains, or low carb, which I have heard are better for you. Before long I am back to eating all kinds of wheat, despite the fact that I know it is not good for me. And all of that because I had not made it a hard rule.

Another example of a hard rule is to make the best choice possible when faced with a craving. I have made it a hard rule to choose only dark chocolate (80% or higher) when I want to eat something sweet. This is important for me because I know that dark chocolate is better for me than a lot of other sweets I could choose. I get the psychological boost from the chocolate, some powerful antioxidants, and very little sugar. You can't say that about ice cream or a sugar cookie. And if you have no dark chocolate in the house, it takes a good bit of effort to go get some, and by that time the craving may be gone.

But be careful here that indulging a craving is something you do on a rare basis, and make that a hard rule too. I allow myself some dark chocolate from time to time as it has been a favorite of mine. Some months go by and I don't eat it. But I do not allow it more than once a month, lest it become a practice that I use to calm myself. If I ate it every day, or even every week it might be something that I would automatically turn to for comfort in times of stress, simply because I had "practiced" it. In fact, it has been a source of comfort for me, even recently, despite the fact that I have recently created a hard rule around it. The idea of chocolate being love is so ingrained in my psyche that I still reach for it when I am using food for comfort. It's important we recognize that no matter how hard we try to control every aspect of our lives, we will still occasionally fall short. We still live in a world where advertising is subtle and invasive and where Temptation wins from time to time. The idea is to get right back to what you know is right for you. Think in larger patterns and longer time frames. Don't waste time lamenting failure and stop beating yourself up. The world does enough of that for us. Just do what is right at the next available opportunity and remember to love yourself for the long term.

I drink coffee every morning. Two to three cups. It is a practice of mine. I recognize that the consistent pattern of drinking it daily means that I am practicing it. However, I have a hard rule when it comes to coffee. I never drink it after noon. A lot of people have that same rule because it keeps them up at night. For a time I was allowing myself a small cup in the afternoon as a pick me up. I was practicing using coffee for increased energy. I was also enjoying it on a psychological level. That may or may not work for you. It didn't work for me in the long term. While in the short term I had more energy I found myself drifting further and further from my hard rule, drinking more and more coffee as each day passed. Soon I was waking up with caffeine withdrawal headaches at 3 am and my stomach was upset at the amount of acid I was taking in. I had to take stock and move back to my hard rule. Within a couple days I was back to what felt more healthy for me.

You might have rituals in your life that aren't as healthy as they could be. Some things are important to us psychologically and we must choose our battles carefully and not to do too much at a time. Today you may be able to stop eating wheat. Maybe in 6 months you will be able to stop drinking diet colas. (Again, these are just examples. I'm not saying these are the right choices for you. This program allows you to study yourself to find out what the scientific evidence says is right for you.)

It is important too, not to simply quit something. You must replace what you quit with something that is better for you. So, if you are going to stop watching television every night, you must replace the behavior with something better. Maybe you take a family walk instead, or play a board game together. Take something inactive and replace it with something fun and active. But before you begin, make a decision to commit to it for a reasonable amount of time. Say you decide to take a month off of TV and replace it with reading books or walks after dinner. For one month you make it a hard rule. After that month reassess. What was it like? Look at the results. Was one month long enough? Maybe you need to do it for six months to see an effect. What positive things came about as a result of the change?

I want to talk about another hard rule I have adopted since beginning to write this book. The hard rule is that I eat mushrooms every single day. It doesn't matter what kind or mushrooms, and as long as I eat the equivalent of 1 medium white button mushroom per day I have met my goal. This is important for me because of two things. First, I have obesity. Second I have a terribly large family history of breast cancer, and cancer in general. You will see in in chapter 9 that mushrooms are very important for both weight loss and maintenance, as well as a cancer preventative and cure. They are so good for us that I am practicing to use mushrooms as a coping food. I generally sauté them with green peppers, onions, and garlic in olive oil spray. I put them in almost everything I eat. For the most part they take on the other flavors of the foods you mix them with, so they are extremely versatile. This mix is a real treat for me, and has all the right earmarks of a healthy and comforting food. Mushrooms are a miracle food that many of us do not eat enough of in America. The details are in Chapter 9, so hang on we will get there!

These are just examples. The point is that you can choose to change your life for the better. You know where you spend your time, what you do for comfort.

Write Your Story

Look at your life and determine what your 'practices' are. What are you doing with your time, day in and day out.

What do you do every single day? What do you do nearly every day?

Write a list of your favorite foods. Be honest! If it is lasagna and garlic bread, it is!

Are these foods truly therapeutic for you?

Do they help in your fight against obesity? Or do they harm your body in the long term?

Make a list of the things you practice daily and weekly.

Now divide that list into things that are therapeutic for you and those which are not healthy practices.

Prioritize the least healthy behaviors/foods and make a plan to get rid of them.

Create one hard rule that will help you to eradicate the worst behavior/food from your life. Write that down and post it somewhere that can be seen by anyone who is in your house. The fridge works well. If you work in an office, post it where you will see it daily. Make it public.

Send an email to your best-ie telling them about your decision and that you need them to help you to be accountable for getting rid of the thing that's causing you harm.

Some people make a pledge to their favorite charity for $5 a week for every week they fail. They give the money to their spouse or a good friend who gives it to the charity when you fail. If you start with $260 in a savings account at the beginning of the year, for example, you can withdraw $5 a week for every week that you fail and turn it over to a charity. If you have success you keep the money. At the end of the year, if you are successful, you will have saved enough money through your behavior to buy a new outfit or something you've been wanting for yourself. Make it more money and maybe you could afford a cruise! Be creative! If you are a smoker, use the money you would have spent on cigarettes to go on a short vacation or buy a guitar!

But choose hard rules, despite the initial pain they may cause you. Be deliberate, tenacious, mindful and use hard rules. You will be much more likely to succeed with a few hard rules than with a whole pack of soft rules.

IDENTITY & HEALTH

Identity. This book is about knowing who you are, and what your identity is. It is about being able to choose that identity, no matter where you begin. It is about being who we want to be. What is your identity? Let's explore identity in general so we're all on the same page. We are a society that all too quickly and way too closely identifies with things, with our jobs, our vocations, our hobbies. We ARE writers and engineers, and mothers or fathers. We ARE political, or apolitical, or painters, or runners, or scrapbookers. It is right there in our language. It should be obvious to us that we are entities separate from what we do. Unfortunately, it is a part of our language and our culture that we take on the identity of what we spend time doing. Further, we speak about almost everything in our lives as though it possesses us.

We ARE fat. What does that mean? If you look at what we are saying, it is clear that we have taken this on as part of our identity. We don't say that we carry around extra weight, or that we HAVE fat, which is probably far more accurate. The really tall, slender guy in class IS lanky. We tend not to separate ourselves from our physical attributes any more than we separate ourselves from what we do.

So who are we? Who are we really? Are we the sum total of the events of our lives? Are we what we do for a living? What is the consequence of identifying so closely with what you do for a living? Think about it; you are at a friend's house for dinner where you meet someone new. Typically in America one of the first questions we ask one another is, "What do you do?" It is an important question because after all we spend a lot of our time at work. It is important because this question tells us a lot about the person, about their interests, their experience and probably something about their educational background and how they live. If for example, the answer is that they are a brick-layer or a hair dresser it tells us that this person works a physically demanding job. It tells us that they are on their feet all day long and gives us an idea of their approximate economic status. After all, we kind of want to know this but are usually too polite to ask directly. Asking what someone does for a living gives us the answer without embarrassing anyone. If on the other hand the answer comes back that they work in intellectual property or artificial intelligence, we can assume a whole host of things about their educational background and that they probably work in an office and that they more than likely make a lot of money. What about the person who is unemployed or underemployed? Often their eyes don't meet ours once we've asked the question "What do you do?" We have basically asked "Who are you?" and sometimes the answer seems to come back, "I'm no one because I do not work". That has been the case for many stay at home mothers for years. These are of course stereotypes and generalizations. But the illustration holds. What we spend our time doing is inextricably linked with our identity. And in many circles some vocations, like staying home with children, aren't valued as highly as working in an office. The conclusion of course is that we don't value people properly. More to the point, we don't value ourselves properly.

What happens when you can no longer do the kind of work that you have for 20 or 30 years? Imagine that your circumstances change overnight. What happens if you are no longer able to do the kind of work you have chosen to identify with for all those years? I imagine that there would be a time of adjustment, maybe even mourning for the loss of that part of our lives. We've all heard the stories of people who retire and just feel lost. What if the unthinkable happens and you are disabled in a way that removes any possibility for work? Or more likely in the current economy, you may get laid off and find it difficult to get another job. There is always an adjustment period and during that time things can get a bit rocky for those around us. Change is difficult, especially life altering change.

It is all about identity. We must discover and then shed those pre-conceived ideas about who we are in order to get to a starting place. It is then that we can re-build our ideal identity. These concepts are so deeply imbedded in our language and culture that unless we address them, we run the risk of unwittingly encouraging the old identity.

What if you lost weight… a lot of weight? That too is a life altering change. But because it is usually a very positive thing, we don't think of it as stressful. I have news for you: all change brings stress. Lasting change brings a higher level of stress for a longer period of time, as we (and those people who love us) adjust.

The reason is that our loved ones are accustomed to our current image, our identity. They know us as the image we have projected to them for years. If we have been fat most of our lives, then our friends and family are accustomed to us being fat. They are comfortable with "who we are" fat and all. Commonly (yes there are rare exceptions) with obesity comes a boatload of emotional baggage. We know this baggage as low self esteem, a lack of self-confidence, poor self-image, and the well worn list could go on. When we get thin it changes us in ways that our family and friends (even we) have probably not anticipated. Not only do we look different, we carry ourselves differently. We gain self-confidence, we improve our outlook on life, and sometimes shed problems like depression. These changes can be very difficult for the people who love us.

The reason these changes are difficult is that all relationships seek balance, just as nature seeks homeostasis. When our relationships balance out, we are at peace with one another. Even if the balance is unhealthy it allows for a certain level of comfort. Unfortunately that comfort is just a form of familiarity. Change that balance, and you upset the equilibrium that gives us comfort in those relationships. But when one or both people are unhealthy the relationship isn't the best it could be for either of them. Familiarity is not enough, especially when someone's health is at risk. That balance must change if the individuals are going to thrive.

Yes, we all think that we want the best for those we people we love. We really do. It is just that sometimes "the best" entails changes that affect us in ways we never anticipated. Be honest with yourself.

How do you feel when your best friend loses weight and you don't? Even if you weren't fat, there is something implied in their weight loss about you. For years you went to the same clubs, but now she gets vastly more attention than when she was fat. That throws off the balance of the relationship. You aren't familiar with this new balance and it can throw you off emotionally.

When I was a kid I was the fat sister. But for five years I was a size 4-6 and it changed the entire balance of the relationships I had with my family of origin. It was uncomfortable to one degree or another for nearly everyone. First, I didn't know how to live without constantly talking about being thin. After all, I had been fat for 40 years! Being thin was one of the most exciting things that had ever happened to me. And I just wanted to roll around in it, enjoy every moment of it. But that gets old for your family and friends who knew you when you actually had something to talk about besides diet and exercise. In many cases this is where they push back. (more on pushback later) Suffice it to say that it is completely understandable that others push back against even our most positive live changes. Change upsets our relationship homeostasis.

Why are we so surprised when we slide back into old comfortable habits including eating too much and exercising too little? It is what we know and it is what others know of us. And after a lifetime of that, it is WHO WE ARE. And although we have changed physically, and we have resisted Temptation and we have better eating patterns and we move a lot more, inside we are still that same person who IS fat. Think about it, when was the last time you saw someone who has been thin all their lives raving endlessly about their great diet and exercise and what size jeans they wear? They don't! They don't because they have taken health and thinness as a part of their identity. Fat people don't get all excited and rave about their day of overconsumption and laying around. It's the same thing.

Here's the multi-million dollar question: how do we truly change WHO WE ARE from fat person to healthy person? That my friend, is the Holy Grail. We know how to diet. We know how to lose weight. The Holy Grail is the more illusive question: How do we keep the weight off forever? The answer is more precious than gold. For at least the last several centuries, scholars the world over haven't been able to answer this question. All the money that is thrown into drug research hasn't touched this problem. If you are reading this you have probably lost and re-gained hundreds of pounds over your lifetime. The good news is, it is not your fault. Until now no one has been able to tell you how to keep the weight off. No one has been able to show you exactly how to have vitality.

This isn't a book that will dictate to you how many cups of broccoli you should eat, or how to jog 30 minutes a day to burn calories. This is a book about learning what works specifically and individually for you. It's about learning what will be successful for you, not every person with your blood type, or even every member in your household.

My husband and I do not do well when we eat the same foods. In the summer time he thrives on a mostly vegetarian diet that is high in carbohydrates, greens and healthy fats. In the winter time he must change his diet to incorporate more fish and starchier vegetables and grains. I do better year round on an anti-inflammation diet that includes low glycemic veggies and a lot of fish. When my husband eats my diet he loses too much weight. When I eat his I gain weight! For years this was a frustration for me. I wanted to make "healthy meals for my family" but was stymied by the results! Nothing was healthy for all of us at the same time! There was always someone in my family who was not thriving in a one size fits all family menu plan. Maybe you will be luckier than I was in this regard and have similar dietary needs within your family. But how do you know? If you are reading this book, it is likely that you are looking for guidance in this area and it may not be clear for you what it means to eat a healthy diet. How you know is by creating your own plan and working through the emotional steps that will keep you on the path to success.

In the past it seemed logical to look to the diet and exercise "experts" for this guidance. But we know from science that these experts have only succeeded with 2% of the population that tries their diet plan. In other words, for most of us, other people's programs don't work for us. We must develop our own program that works specifically for us. You are an expert on you. Let's use that. It's the only way to be sure you will have success.

This book is a process of discovery, if you will allow it. It is meant to guide you to find out who you really are, and how to change who you are for the better. It is not easy. It will take some work on your part. But I promise you that if you do the work you will understand more about yourself and how to create and live authentically with vitality within the identity and the body you have always wanted.

WHITE KNUCKLING IT

Are you ready? I am not asking if you are ready to lose weight. This isn't about will-power, and it isn't about white knuckling it. That's old school weight loss and you know it doesn't work. You know as well as I do that you can only white knuckle it for so long until you have to let go. What happens when you let go? You crash. Again. If successful weight loss was just a matter of calories in and calories out, we would have solved this problem many decades ago.

This is about change. Lasting, life long change.

Life long change ruffles feathers. What I mean by that is some of your relationships will be enhanced by the changes you make to your identity during this process. Some however, will dissolve. I firmly believe that if you change from unhealthy to healthy in mind and in body and your Friday night pizza binge buddy doesn't change with you, there will be friction… a lot of friction. If someone really cares about you they will always want the long term best for you. They will keep your best interests as a priority. I can say un-categorically that a Friday night pizza binge (or any binge) is not in your best interests. We all have people in our lives who can be a lot of fun but they aren't always a good influence on us.

My point is, are you ready to change those relationships that aren't good for you? Are you ready to talk with those folks honestly about the harmful things that you do together? This isn't a blame session - you made these choices too. It is possible that your binge buddy wants out as bad as you do, but loves spending time with you. You can change what you do together to reflect who you are, who you want to be, who you are becoming. It may end up that you just spend less time with that person. But your change means change for everyone you know.

It might be as simple as something you and your partner buy

together that isn't good for you. It took me a surprisingly long time to tell my partner that corn chips were a real weakness for me. It was hard on a couple levels. First, they are a weakness for me, so naturally I didn't want to let them go. Second, I know he likes them. I didn't want to deprive him of something he likes. Well, to my surprise, when I finally came out with my confession, it was no big deal. He immediately jumped to support me and we haven't bought chips of any kind since then. When you tell someone who loves you that something is a stumbling block for you, that ought to be the response. It's not always, but your approach is important. If you approach it as a plea for help rather than a blame game, it seems to me your chances of success are much higher.

It is possible that you don't have a binge buddy at all. A lot of people hide what they eat from the people who know them. They hide in large and small ways. It's not always the secret runs through the drive through. People have said to me, "I don't see why you are overweight at all! You hardly eat anything!" I'm pretty sure that they never saw me eat in front of the TV with a full plate of spaghetti on my chest! It wasn't pretty.

The deck is really stacked against those of us who suffer from the disease of obesity. You don't have to binge eat, or overeat at all if your genes dictate that you store energy more readily than others. In my family we called ourselves "The Famine People" because if we had been born in a different time in history or a different place in the world, we would be the lucky ones. We store so much energy that we could literally survive a famine, and yet today in America and much of the world we have tons of food (and food like substances) all around us every day. The big problem with being of the Famine People Clan is that there is also an internal drive to eat whenever food is present, as if our next meal won't happen for days. It takes some real self-awareness for Famine People to stop and think before eating a meal that our next meal will only be four hours away and that the calories we are consuming only have to fuel us for those four hours. Understand that if you want to be your ideal, if you want to live your best, most authentically healthy life, you must choose it. Above all, you must be ready to choose to be true to yourself, not to your binge buddy, not to anyone else's vision of what you should be.

If you have obesity, you are probably (like me) a member of the Famine People Clan. You are in good company. Despite the stereotypes of fat people, you should understand what our group really looks like, statistically anyway. Keep in mind, these are in a way generalizations too. But they are based in research, not personal prejudices. First, we will look at reality.

Stereotypes hold that people with obesity are lazy, untrustworthy, not conscientious, jolly, funny, ugly, mentally unstable, unproductive, liars, prone to exaggeration, uninformed, uneducated, stupid, slow, you know the list. Nothing could be further from the truth. Yes, there is a small minority of people like that. That is how stereotypes begin. But research shows that people with the disease of obesity are as varied as anyone with any other disease. One researcher has three categories of people with obesity, the smallest of which is a very small group of mentally unstable people. This percentage is on par with the general public, statistically. In other words, there are no more mentally unstable people with obesity than there are in the general public. The largest category (highest percentage) of people with obesity are characterized by van der Merwe (2007) as being extroverts who are very talented, with a good sense of reality and body image, and who also happen not to be able to resist the social cues around them that suggest they should eat.

In terms of personality types, we the Famine People are a normal cross section of society too. That means we are pretty much the same as the general population in terms of our identities. We are all different, and we are overweight for different reasons. During this important journey, you will discover why you have this incurable disease called obesity.

I've said that phrase a few times now and I want to explain it a bit. It is very important that you understand that if you are chronically overweight, obese, or even what is called super (or morbidly) obese, you have a disease. This disease is incurable. That is important.

Most people who are overweight think that when they diet and lose the weight the problem is solved; the disease is cured. If you have ever read a diet book, that's probably where you got that notion. That is WRONG. Obesity is a life long, incurable disease. You must manage this disease for the rest of your life. It is no different than if you had a thyroid disorder or diabetes. These diseases do not go away just because your blood levels look normal. You must continue to take your medications and blood levels in order to manage these diseases. All too often diet gurus calling themselves experts base their "programs" on their own experiences, or the anecdotal experiences of a handful of loyal followers. Even more dangerous, there is of late a new type of "expert" in the field that you should be aware of. Do not be taken in by the self-proclaimed experts who have hired Investigator-Sponsored Research Companies to verify their claims. Admittedly, it is really hard to know if a guru has done this. Difficult, but not impossible. These "experts" will typically hire a company that exists for the sole purpose of doing research that some how "proves" that the products or programs of these "experts" really work. Most gurus who create programs are simply not testing them at all. They rely for the most part on word of mouth marketing (no longer just a natural phenomenon) and testimonials.

The first thing that diet gurus do is to tell you what they are proposing you spend money on is NOT A DIET! And make no mistake friend, they ALL require you spend money on their program, website, software, and products. They are in business. The diet business. Ok, but let's define that term and talk about what a real diet is and what the word 'diet' has come to mean in our culture. First, you must know by now that what the guru is trying to do by denying their program is a diet, is to differentiate themselves from the crowd of other diet gurus out there. They just want to seem different in order to get your attention. And dieting has a bad reputation in our culture and has become synonymous with suffering. So, no one wants that next to their name. For the record, what a diet really is, and I know that you know this, is a way of eating. Simple as that. Google Dictionary says, "A special course of food to which one restricts oneself, either to lose weight or for medical reasons." If what the diet gurus are offering is not a diet, I do not know what it is. Simply put a diet by any other name (lifestyle, for example) is still a diet.

I happen to see a personal trainer's reality TV show the other day and it was amazing to me that he kept telling the woman he was training things like "you've got to get out of your own way" and "you can do this!" and "you are capable of so much more" and "you need to be comfortable with being uncomfortable". All these platitudes mean nothing if you can't tell the person HOW TO DO IT. Over and over again I see this kind of thing. The worst part is hearing the trainee telling her trainer with all earnestness, "I know I can do better. It just means that I have to be perfect every day, day in and day out." There is no guidance, no emotional or psychological process that could get those people to their goal without looking forward to a life of white knuckling it. And that is in a nutshell why diets and fitness programs fail long term. You can't succeed on just platitudes. They can only sustain you for a short time, and since you haven't made a real lasting psychologically life altering change, you will be forced to live your trainer's life. Not your own. It works for your trainer because that is their identity. They have made these platitudes meaningful for their lives. And while it works for them, organic change by-proxy doesn't work for you.

Until you come through your own psychological change, you will never be able to stop white knuckling it. You will feel like you have to hold your breath constantly because if you ever let a breath out, your whole world would tumble in on you. Fitness by-proxy, diet by-proxy, change by-proxy doesn't work.

All I mean by those terms is that when you take someone else's fitness plan, or diet plan and try to apply it to your own life, all you get is mimicry. You are simply mimicking someone else's successful behavior. That would be ok, if it worked. It doesn't.

It is like learning to play an instrument when you are a kid. First, you must mimic the teacher in how she holds her hands on the instrument, how she blows into the horn. You do it, and a sort of familiar sound comes out. But becoming a musician is a much more personal, in depth experience. It comes after years of mimicry of a teacher's methods until finally you can create your own sounds and your own style, and it is only when you can finally "own" your instrument and really make your own unique, beautifully flowing sounds, that you can say that you are a musician.

We have spent decades mimicking fitness and diet gurus in what works for them. We don't listen to our bodies. We do things that are dangerous to our health and wellbeing and maybe for a time we are thinner. But we are still only copying what that teacher has shown us. We've accomplished no real change in our lives.

I've seen people mimic Weight Watchers for years at a time, and they keep the weight off for that time. But if they ever miss a meeting the white knuckling begins.

I saw an interesting discussion on Facebook the other day. The young woman was asking about the latest diet trend, "the cheat day". I was interested in what people thought about that so I read the thread. The heart of the argument is that when people allow themselves a cheat day, or a cheat meal, they are more likely to stay on a diet plan for longer.

What this amounts to is that it breaks up your white knuckling with days on which you can relax and be yourself. That makes white knuckling easier. Do you realize how crazy that sounds? Who are you cheating? When you "cheat" on a diet, you are literally only cheating yourself. The diet doesn't care if you cheat. The diet guru doesn't care- they already have your money.

What you are doing is pouring something that is bad for you into your body. Any diet that necessitates you occasionally putting something bad into your body isn't for you. If you feel the need to cheat just to get through the week, you haven't changed a thing. It's the difference between going on a two week vacation or moving to another country. If you are white knuckling at all, you are on a vacation. You haven't made a real life change.

This book is about change. It is about you becoming who you need to be in order to become whole, healthy, and authentic. Spending your life white knuckling means that you are desperately holding on to something that isn't yours.

You MUST find what will work for you- every day 24/7 and 365 days a year for the rest of your life. Not something that worked for a celebrity. You have no idea the reality behind why their program worked for them.

I was thinking about the television reality show, The Biggest Loser. Fun tv that does a lot of good for a few people and inspires the rest of us. But a lot goes on behind the scenes of the tv show that the viewers never see. The physical therapy, specialized workout recovery tools and equipment, massage and physical therapists, doctors monitoring and treating the contestants daily and tending to injuries resulting from over exercising. After all working out for four to six hours a day takes a toll on the human body, especially if you have to carry a lot of extra weight.

And although they sell workout videos and games, inspirational books and cookbooks, they still miss the point. A lot of their success lies in the fact that they assign personal trainers, producers and camera people to follow contestants around 24/7 making sure that they comply with the rules, in many cases screaming at them, guilting them, manipulating them, or just pleading with them when they don't. And for many contestants this works, while they are under that kind of scrutiny. How could that possibly translate long term to the average person?

The short answer is that it doesn't translate long term. It doesn't translate because it isn't internal change. These are externally motivated changes that don't stick when the external motivation is not longer there.

Don't get me wrong, The Biggest Loser TV show seems to have honorable motives and they do a lot of good in terms of feeding the hungry and inspiring people to do better for themselves. But inspiration is only a tiny tiny part of the process. It's the part that gets you interested in change. That's it.

You will see later in the book why this makes sense.

Write Your Story

How would you describe yourself?

When you first meet someone, what is it that they learn first about you?

What is the first impression you give to others?

In 2 sentences or less, who are you?

Who do you admire?

If you could live a life like someone else does, whose life would you live? Why?

What do you like about yourself most?

List your best qualities.

What would you change about yourself? Why?

What habits do you have that are good for you?

How do you feel about your job? Why?

How would your boss describe you?

How would your best friend describe you?

How would the person in your life who is most critical of you (who is not you) describe you?

List 5 habits related to health that you would like to see incorporated into your life.

What motivates you to change? Are these internal motivations? or external?

List three internal motives for changing to a healthier life.

WHAT SHOULD I EAT?

This is by far the most common question I get. We have been conditioned by the diet industry to be told what to eat, how, when, and where to eat it. We've been force-fed pre-prepared meals, liquid diets, and pills. "Eat bacon... wait don't eat bacon!" "Coffee is good for you... oops! Now it isn't.... Ok, maybe it is." Nutrition is by far one of the most confusing and widely reported subjects in media reports. It is in the media every day. Every day there is news about what and how to eat. Yet no two experts agree! How is the average everyday person supposed to get up in the morning and know that the dietary choices they make every day are the right ones? It's a bit like foraging in the woods for mushrooms. Unless you are a mycologist (mushroom expert), you probably shouldn't be making those choices. Some mushrooms are poisonous! I wouldn't last a day! Yet here we are, ordinary people with no specific education about nutrition, picking our own foods! Yikes! Watch out for poisonous mushrooms!

And I have said this before, but I will say it again. I am not a medical doctor. I am not a nutritionist, or dietician. I am a research psychologist who is focused on a real cure for obesity. That has led me to study nutrition, exercise, and more importantly the psychological processes that are involved in obesity, weight loss, and weight gain. So, this chapter is really just my musings, observations, and a distillation of my own education based on the research of others.

Diet is necessary, but not sufficient.

I have one rule for myself. That's it. Just the one. I ask this question each time I eat, and I try to be mindful enough to do it every time I eat. This is the question:

Is what I am about to eat as nutritious as it could possibly be?

That's it.

Eat good food and don't eat bad food. Sounds easy, doesn't it?

What is good food and what is bad food? I think this is a little like the Supreme Court's definition of pornography: You know it when you see it. It doesn't take a panel of experts to decide that apples are good food. You know it instinctively. Yes, the issue is more complex than that. Of course it is. That complexity is based largely on the individual's co-morbidities and nutritional requirements. For example, if you are diabetic, an apple may not be as good for you as say a cup of cooked lentils or peanut butter. It is up to you to know your body, know about food, listen to your body, your doctors, and to be responsible for your choices. To review the info on co-morbidities, jump back to chapter four by clicking here. Or resume reading...

The less processed your food, the better it is for you. The closer you get to the beginning of the food chain and the closer you get to something you could grow in your own back yard, the more nutritional value that food will have. It is that simple. When you eat for nutrition, the calorie issue will resolve itself. Foods higher in nutrients are (for the most part) lower in calories. That makes it very simple!

I think that the rule we have been taught to follow is "How can I make this taste as good as it can taste?" When did dinner start requiring 'excitement'? Advertising from the food industry doesn't have our best interests in mind. They have profit in mind. Not your health. Take for example the ads from the Corn Grower's Association defending High Fructose Corn Syrup (HFCS). The message is clear: HFCS is the same as sugar and your body can't tell the difference. Ask any biologist or neurologist if there is a difference between HFCS and sugar, you will get a distinctly different answer from what's in the Corn Industry commercial. HFCS is highly concentrated and it is TOXIC especially if you have obesity or diabetes. In 2010 Princeton researchers found that HFCS prompts considerably more weight gain than table sugar. In fact, in the Princeton study, no weight was gained from sugar, but HFCS (and equal calorie intake) meant a considerable weight gain in the rats they tested.

Along the same lines of food products that encourage weight gain is MSG. As an obesity researcher I have learned that researchers who study rats and the various issues of obesity have to do something before they can begin. They must make their "rat test subjects" fat. Rats typically do not get fat on their own. It's tough to do research on obese rats when there simply are so few found in nature!

To that end, it is a common practice to feed research rats MSG pellets. This is the most effective way to make rats fat in the shortest amount of time. WOW! Let that sink in. That is not the experiment. It is simply a way to prepare thin rats to become fat rats upon which we can experiment.

Consider now that most processed foods contain MSG which can act as both a flavor enhancer and as preservative. Wow, it has to be way cheaper to use a flavor enhancer that also preserves the food it is enhancing! No wonder companies use it! But this is important: if you are buying a prepared meal that is chicken flavored, it probably has literally no chicken (no chicken broth, no chicken fat, etc.) in it. Turns out that the savory flavor of chicken is well mimicked by MSG. And MSG is far cheaper than actual chicken. Never mind that it isn't chicken, maybe you can live with that. What you cannot afford to live with, if you have obesity, is that you are eating a substance that is known to cause weight gain.

It is commonly found in Asian food, even just stir fried veggies and rice will have it. And now even these "mom and pop" restaurants are hip to those of us who do not want it in our diets. They tell us very often that they do not ADD MSG to their food. There is a good chance that is true. They might not be ADDING MSG to their food as they prepare it. But even if it is true, many of these restaurants still buy their sauces and specialty oils pre-made and those very often contain MSG. So, while the Asian food restaurant owner isn't ADDING MSG to the food they make, they very often are adding sauces and oils that contain it. You may even see this careful wording on prepared food labels. It is just one more way to make the consumer think they are getting something without MSG, when there is MSG in it. MSG is a naturally occurring compound, make no mistake. But just because it is naturally occurring, that doesn't mean it is good for you. The same holds true with the "no sugar added" label. While ice cream can be no sugar added, it still contains milk sugars in abundance and maybe even HFCS! Read the nutrient label, not just the front of the box.

Just one last thing about MSG and HFCS: These terrible ingredients have many many different names. You just about have to be a chemist to know them all! And the food industry keeps adding and changing the names they use and the various ways that they can legally represent these toxic substances. (Click on the word 'names' above to read an article about some of the many names of MSG.) Just a small sample of the article: "MSG can hide under the names sodium caseinate or calcium caseinate and even under natural-sounding names, such as bouillon, broth stock, or malt extract." (From Livestrong.org) Even the innocent sounding "natural flavorings" is MSG!

Concentrated Food Is Dangerous

All processed foods are concentrated in one way or another. Why is that important? It is important because the same volume of food will cost you far far more calories when it is concentrated than when it is whole, fresh or raw. If you process food it becomes super condensed. Anyone who has ever made a blueberry pie knows this. Even if you haven't made a blueberry pie but just eaten one, you can clearly see it. The fruit in the pie (now unrecognizable) has been squished and boiled down to a liquid form with a lot of added sugar and who knows what else to preserve it. Then we add some fancy stuff to make it stiff enough to sit up on our plates and put it into a crust.

Eating blueberries is a much different experience from eating blueberry pie. One experience is much healthier than the other. Hazard a guess? It isn't difficult to see that eating fresh blueberries is much more nutritious than eating blueberry pie. And because the pie is concentrated you will likely eat many more berries and a whole lot of other ingredients (including lard- don't get me started) and calories than you would if you simply ate the berries. What's more, the berries lose a great deal of their nutrients when they are cooked as they are for the pie. Further, the concentrated sugar and lack of nutrients causes your body to want to eat more and more of it because what you are craving is the missing nutrition! Your brain recognizes via your taste buds that you are eating blueberries, but somehow you are not getting the same nutrients that you expect from eating raw, fresh, blueberries. So you keep looking for nutrients in the pie. After several slices you are finally "full" but amazingly still not satisfied.

What is most important about our food choices? Does what we choose fulfill the nutrient needs of our bodies? If that is your concern, as it is mine, you will make the best choices you can for your body. You have to ask yourself when you are about to pull into a drive thru, "What is the most nutritious thing I can eat?" Maybe it is a salad. Maybe the answer is to turn away from the drive thru and into the grocery store parking lot a block away and buy a bag of carrots.

I talk a lot about raw plant food, but I am a pragmatist. There are two vegetables: carrots and celery, that increase in anti-oxidant value when you cook them- and pretty much no matter how you cook them. They do lose enzymatic action when cooked, but the increase in vitamins may be enough to sway me to cook them now and again.

Diet is important. It is necessary. But if it were sufficient, the obesity problem would not be an epidemic. The problem is now so wide spread that the World Health Organization calls the problem "Globesity". All but the poorest underdeveloped nations of the world have this problem.

The problem is that very often we don't eat just for hunger or nutrition. We eat to celebrate, we eat to mourn, for comfort or because we are bored. We eat for about as many reasons as there are people on earth! But some of us have a disease. We have the incurable disease of obesity. And this disease demands that we manage it, every day and for the rest of our lives. That's a long tough road. My goal in all of this is to give you insights and tools that will help make managing this disease easier for you. And once you have navigated the eight stages in this book, I am confident that your decisions will have more staying power than you ever dreamed possible.

Medical issues are important too. It is widely understood that having obesity creates risks for many other diseases like type 2 diabetes, coronary heart disease, hypertension, sleep apnea, gallbladder disease, and certain types of cancer (Echols, 2010; Mehler, Lasater, & Padilla, 2003; Stewart et al., 2010). This is well understood. What isn't as widely known or understood are pain syndromes that come with having obesity. Inflammation also accompanies obesity and where there is inflammation, there is pain. Obesity is a very painful disease! It causes pain and swelling in your joints, and inflammation in connective tissues, which all lead to the body breaking down over time. Inflammation may very well be at the root of all human age related diseases (Weil, 2012).

Eating a 50% raw whole food diet that contains no red meat, industrially processed foods, or animal byproducts like cheese, commercially processed eggs, wheat, gluten, or milk can help decrease your inflammation and as a result, pain. In addition, avoiding nightshade vegetables and citrus fruits has been found to help with inflammation. But you really must test these ideas to see what works for your body. I have found that some of this wisdom is very helpful for me, some of it doesn't seems to push my inflammatory markers up at all.

An interesting thing happens when you eat more than 50% cooked food. You body reacts to the food in much the same way that it reacts to a cut or infection. It produces inflammation to combat it. In order to balance that out and avoid adding inflammation to your already over-burdened body, you should try to eat at least half your daily intake as raw whole fruits, veggies, nuts, seeds, or gluten free grains. You can include dried fruit because the definition of raw food is anything not cooked over 117 degrees (104 if you are really strict). Dehydrated foods qualify as raw.

A little secret: raw whole foods (by and large) have very high nutrient levels and very low calorie counts.

When you cook foods you damage or remove enzymes that help with digestion, not to mention losing a lot of the vitamins and minerals. And check this out for yourself, but I find that the more raw food I eat, the better I feel. (you know I'm not talking about raw meat, right?)

It's not an easy way to eat initially, so I recommend starting with 80% cooked foods, 20% raw whole foods. Change by 10% a week until you reach 50-50. And try to get your oils from eating whole foods like avocado, seeds, nuts, or lightly processed olives. These suggestions are interesting, but remember no one diet works for everyone. It is vital that you find out for yourself what works for you. These are just options for you to think about testing for yourself.

Some people suffer from gas when they begin to eat a lot of raw food. For me an over the counter anti-gas product removed the symptoms. Eventually, my body got used to the diet and the excess gas went away. Make no mistake, if you eat meat and dairy products, your body went through a similar adjustment period. Most of us do not remember it because we began eating these things as children. I have read that the natural norm for our bodies is being lactose intolerant, but we have eaten dairy for so many generations we actually think of lactose intolerance as a disorder!

A word about dairy and meat consumption is in order. It is important you understand what works for you. I am not asking you to become a raw foodie or a vegetarian or a vegan. I will recommend some things for you to try that I think are in your best interest and in the best interest of the planet. But if eating meat works for you, then eat meat. This program will provide you with a way to determine exactly what is best for your body, your energy levels, moods, productivity, etc. Do not simply mimic me. That is of little value to you and no better than following any of a million diet gurus.

Heart disease is the number one medical killer in America, and in many other developed nations. Whether you agree or disagree with it, there is a literal ton of evidence that supports the link between cholesterol and heart disease. By the same token, there is a literal ton of research that links inactivity and heart disease. Cholesterol is a substance that your body produces, and that you get more of when you eat animal products. You cannot raise your cholesterol levels without ingesting animal products. Some of us make too much cholesterol on our own without eating meat. Certainly, if you eat meat your cholesterol numbers will be higher than if you do not eat meat, fish, eggs, and dairy. This is almost an oversimplification, but I think there is a lot we do not know about this issue, and I am not a biochemist or a medical doc. The quality of the animal products is vitally important in this equation. Corn fed beef has such a natural ring to it! It sounds very healthy, doesn't it? But cows are not vegetarians. Cows are herbivores. They live on grass, not vegetables like corn. Feed a cow corn (or anything but grass) and you must compensate for that choice by also feeding the cow medicines that stop their stomachs from exploding from gas! That's part of the reason our beef supply has so many antibiotics! Corn is cheaper than grass land. American corn subsides have made it so much cheaper that it is still cheaper when you include anti-gas remedies and antibiotics! It's bad for the cow's health and bad for our health. It is only good for the beef industry and profit.

However, there are many benefits of eating grass fed beef in terms of cholesterol levels. Grass fed beef has much more beneficial omega fats than corn fed beef. There is evidence that it doesn't raise cholesterol levels as a result. Grass-based diets have been shown to enhance total conjugated linoleic acid (CLA) (C18:2) isomers, trans vaccenic acid (TVA) (C18:1 t11), a precursor to CLA, and omega-3 (n-3) FAs on a g/g fat basis (Daley, Abbott, Doyle, Nader & Larson, 2010; Leheska, Thompson, Howe, Hentges, Boyce, Brooks, & Miller, 2008).

From my perspective, the diseases that I have, including obesity call for me to make changes in my diet that will reduce my risk of further diseases and help me manage obesity too. I (as you know by now) have RA, which is an inflammatory autoimmune disease. Animal flesh must be cooked or processed to be eaten safely. The more cooked food I eat, the more inflammation my body produces. That is true, by the way for most people whether you have an inflammatory disease or not. Obesity is also an inflammation producing disease. So, if you have obesity, you have inflammation. And I want to do everything I can do to reduce and limit the amount of inflammation I have in my body. It just makes sense. Look into it for yourself. Get your doc (Naturopathic docs are a great resource for this) on board to help by ordering blood tests to confirm that what you are doing is working.

Beyond the inflammation issue, I have a strong family history of cancer. It runs in my family like it's in line at a Black Friday Sale! Both biological parents have had cancer, and one sibling too. This is another health concern for people with obesity because many many studies link obesity to breast, colon and ovarian cancers.

What is important to me in all this is that I err on the side of protecting my health. Eventually you will deal with your choices in life. One way or another. Eating things that are not the best foods you can eat will eventually turn on you and ravage your body. I'm not saying that there is a list of foods that everyone should avoid at all costs. What I am saying is that you must find out for sure how your body is responding to your food choices.

There seems to be a united battle cry for our "desperate need" for protein. We tend to forget that greens, beans, nuts, grains, and seeds all have protein. Even fruit has a little protein. We are so ill-educated that we think that we have enormous needs for protein, when in fact, a balanced diet with plenty of protein (bioavailable protein) requires no meat at all.

This notion of bioavailability is an important one. It's not about what you eat. It's about how much of the nutrients from that food get into your blood stream. Meat is not an efficient bioavailable food source, although this is controversial depending upon the quality of meat. The problems that come with eating a lot of meat are immense. High protein diets are linked to cancer and of course corn fed beef is linked to increases in blood cholesterol. One problem is that it takes a lot longer to digest meat and during that time nutrients are lost, and decomposing begins. This gives our bodies fewer of the nutrients and more time for the toxins to be absorbed into our intestines. More important than all that to those of us who struggle with excess fat and weight is that adding low quality foods that contain a high saturated fat count to your diet is counterproductive.

Here are a few (albeit extreme) examples:

A 6 oz. porterhouse steak (which is small by porterhouse standards) may have 36 grams of protein, but with it you will be ingesting 44 grams of fat, 16 of them saturated. A 10 oz. Porterhouse has about 67 grams of protein, it also has between 62 and 98 grams of fat depending upon marbling!

That's a minimum of 562 calories from fat alone! Add to all that over 100% of the daily recommended amount of dietary cholesterol.

Here's a head scratcher: Why is there ANY daily recommendation for cholesterol intake? It is not a nutrient.

References: U.S. Department of Agriculture: Search the USDA National Nutrient Database for Standard Reference.

Meanwhile, a 6 oz. portion of soybeans offers a complete protein (amino acid profile) has 72.98 grams of protein, but less than 12 grams of fat, only 1 gram of it saturated, no cholesterol, and 197 mg of calcium, among a lot of other nutrients. Let's be real. No plant food contains cholesterol. I was just reading the nutrient values for spinach that claimed spinach was "very low in cholesterol". In fact, Spinach has no cholesterol. This is true of all plant foods. I hate it when I see an advertisement for a food that never had cholesterol and it says, "No Cholesterol!" as if the food company did something to make it cholesterol free.

FDA approved a soy health claim in 1999 that states that 25 grams of soy protein a day as part of a diet low in saturated fat and cholesterol may reduce the risk of heart disease. That is about two servings of soy foods per day but varies on products used. Foods that meet the labeling must have at least 6.25 g soy protein/serving. And on the environmental side, soybeans can produce 5 to 10 times more protein per acre than land set aside for grazing animals to make milk, and up to 15 times more protein per acre than land set aside for meat production.

I could have compared lower fat beef options or even fish options, but I could have chosen different beans to compare as well.

Soy isn't the only star of the bean world in nutritional terms either. I chose the most controversial, highest fat bean I could find to compare to meat. If I were to do a comparison to lentils, for example, we would see that one cup of cooked lentils contains 18 grams of protein, about 1 gram of fat, no saturated fat at all, no cholesterol, and 37% of the iron you need each day. Soy is controversial, and you might need to take into account your own risks for things like breast cancer when deciding to include it in your diet.

The lowest fat percentage I could find in beef, for example was 95%, leaving 5% fat content. That translates to 6 grams of fat, 3 saturated, and 67 mg of cholesterol in 100 grams of cooked hamburger. Still no contest. Veggies, fruits, nuts, seeds and grains dominate for nutritional value and health benefits, especially for people with obesity.

People who suffer from obesity must know and pay close attention to these important facts. They must know their own numbers.

More and more body builders and other athletes are moving to a plant based diet because of the bioavailability of vegetables and legumes. Spinach is 30% protein and no fat, 56% vitamin A, and a cup is only 7 calories.

The focus of all of this is that we should want to hedge our bets on the side of not adding to our risk of disease. We already have some risk by simply being a person who inflicted with obesity.

Our motivation for losing weight has to be rooted and grounded in our desire for a healthy body.

If all you want is to be "skinny" and look like a model (who is impossible to replicate because of common techniques like air brushing photos) then this is not the book for you. There are plenty of others out there who will serve you better. But the more important motivation you must have is to have a healthier mind. Psychological health is just as important as physical health but we do not emphasize things that we can't see and or touch in Western cultures. It is relatively easy to hide your unhealthy thinking and habits. But that is not an authentic integrated healthy life.

The goal of this book is to get you (and me) closer to living an authentic, healthy life. That means that as your body gets healthier, your mind follows suit or vise versa.

How will we do this? Throughout this book there will be exercises that you can do and repeat as needed. Anyone who has ever seen a nutritionist or a dietician has gone through the experience of the Food Journal. This process is similar. We will do a type of food journal, but with some important twists. We will keep track of energy, productivity, mood, and a host of other items that can help bring us closer to who we want to be.

One of my bad food triggers is comfort. For years when I needed comfort I would go to KFC and get a chicken meal for the whole family. Potatoes, gravy, biscuits, and of course lots of chicken. Forget the green beans. Give me the other stuff. It was so obvious a pattern that anytime I was crying my sweet husband would say something like, "Do you want me to stop at KFC?" He just wanted to make me feel better, and he knew that was one thing that worked. But it only worked in the short term.

True confession: by getting a meal for the whole family I was better able to disguise my own huge portions. I'm pretty sure they knew how much I was eating. But I had myself fooled into thinking they didn't.

Once I became aware of why I was craving KFC when I was

stressed out, I was able make better choices. I chose this food, by the way, because some of the happiest times when I was a kid were spent with my family on little KFC picnics. I may be mistaken, but I think my sisters have had this same knee jerk reaction to stress from time to time.

But that level of analysis is just level one. Simple stuff. You've heard it all before. It is easy to record what you eat, and figure out what it means to you. Why do you have the routines you have? Starting now we are going to go deeper and deeper into those routines and habits and get to the root of why we have this nasty disease.

Listen to your body first. Weigh everything you read/see/hear with what your body says to you. Your body may be sensitive to a diet high in fiber. You may have to very gradually change your diet over time to include more raw fruits and vegetables. Maybe you have iron poor blood and need to take iron supplements until you are no longer anemic. Talk to your doctor about your co-morbidities. Ask how the other diseases or conditions you have are effecting your obesity and vise versa. Ask how your medications are affecting your obesity. Many medications do have an effect on your ability to lose weight and some have a weight gain effect. That's not an excuse.

A lot of Americans are on anti-depressant medications. These meds save lives. No doubt in my mind. I am among the list of people for whom this is true. I'm SO thankful for the meds that gave me back my life! But they also have the unfortunate side effect of weight gain. Talk to your doctor and psychologist or psychiatrist about this if you are concerned. Sometimes these meds are needed during a rough patch in a person's life. Some people need them for life. Know which kind of person you are and if long term anti-depressants are appropriate for you or not. Do not stop taking medications without first consulting your physician, specifically the physician who prescribed them. First, it is not wise to quit many medications of this nature cold turkey. Secondly, you may need to be on them! A thinner body is no good if you are suicidal! I promise you that we can do many things to work with and around these meds!

I have had both depression and fibromyalgia, for which I take Cymbalta. Cymbalta is one of those meds that can cause weight gain. This is frustrating for sure! If you are like me in this, stay tuned! There are some very exciting things coming up that can help you, even if you have to take these meds long term like I do!

A Word About Diet Sodas

*Diet soda consumption in our culture is crazy! And at least one reason for that is many of us have bought into the idea that it is a guilt-free treat. It IS NOT! What aspartame or sucralose together with caffeine do in the brain is to stimulate your appetite, increase carbohydrate cravings, kill brain cells, and maybe worst of all for us they stimulate fat storage and increase weight gain.

Splenda, which has been touted as very safe because it is made from sugar, is in fact very dangerous!

*Studies have revealed that sucralose can cause:

- Shrinking of the thymus glands

- Enlarged liver and kidneys

- Atrophy of lymph follicles in the spleen and thymus

- Reduced growth rate

- Decreased red blood cell count

- Diarrhea

*Aspartame can trigger or worsen the following diseases:

- Multiple sclerosis

- Epilepsy

- Chronic fatigue syndrome

- Parkinson's disease

- Alzheimer's disease

- Mental retardation

- Lymphoma

- Birth defects

- Fibromyalgia

- Diabetes

(*Information provided by ForksOverKnives.com For more information watch the documentary "Forks Over Knives" or check their website: http://www.hungryforchange.tv/are-diet-sodas-making-us-fat)

Now that you know all that, you have to ask yourself if what you are doing habitually the best you can do for your body? Are you practicing good health? Is what you are eating the most nutritious thing you can put into my body? In terms of soda pop I think there are a lot of alternatives that are better. I used to think that stevia was an excellent natural zero calorie sweetener. After all, it is natural and you can grow it in your back yard. But for some people, like me, who are allergic to ragweed and grasses, stevia can be toxic! It has cause my liver counts to skyrocket on a couple occasions before I realized what the issue was. And be sure that if you are going to eat stevia that you watch labels carefully because it is often processed with aspartame or sucralose which you don't want to ingest if you can help it. Sometimes it is processed with rice in order to control portions as it is very sweet and can become bitter when too much is used.

I like foods whose names I can pronounce. And I like to eat things that, if the climate was right, I could grow them in my back yard. Those are all signs that what you are eating is probably better than something created in a test tube. (Obviously, not all natural things that you can grow in your yard are good for you to eat. Poison mushrooms are not good. Arsenic and ricin are both found in nature but you should never eat them as they are deadly.) I think you get the bigger point about things you can grow versus food like substances that have been processed industrially.

It is a lot easier than you think to make and eat raw food. I have been doing it for some time. The following video is from Food Matters, and it shows you in a couple minutes how easy it is to make your own almond milk, for example. I wanted to share this because that was one of those products I never thought in a million years would be this easy!

The Importance of B12 For Vegans

Vitamin B12 regulates brain function, red blood cell production and is essential for life. You cannot live without it! For those of us who fight obesity, it is also incredibly important in the synthesis of fatty acids and the production of energy! If you are tired of being tired, try B12. It is water based, which means you don't have to worry about over dosing. What your body doesn't need will be eliminated during urination. A friend once complained of having "very high priced urine" and I have to say that I would rather have high priced urine than a high priced doctor bill! B12 is not expensive! You can get it a number of ways, all under $10. I like the sublingual form, but you can get liquid forms and pill forms. I also take it in my daily B Complex. It's that important to the fight against obesity. Lack of B12 can lead to nerve damage, anemia, depression, and stomach problems.

For a long time I thought that the only plentiful food borne source of the vitamin B12 is through ingesting animal products. This is a nutrient you need every day. There is one vegetarian B12 source I have just been made aware of and that is miso soup. This Asian breakfast tradition contains a world of great nutrients! It has a good amount of calcium, magnesium, vitamins A & E and is high in isoflavones and protective fatty acids. It can be found in most health food stores, but be sure that when you buy it prepackaged it does not contain MSG (and remember there are many names for MSG). The bacteria in miso synthesizes B12 which is great news for vegans. If you have the disease of obesity, or the family heritage that would predispose you to obesity or heart disease, it is a far better trade off to have to take a little B12 each day than to eat a high fat and cholesterol filled diet in order to get it. B12 isn't just a good idea. This is vitally important. If you choose a vegan diet, be sure to take a high quality B12 supplement or eat miso soup in order to meet those needs. Ask your doctor about B12.

Some people argue that because a plant based diet cannot give you every nutrient you need- (although with the addition of miso to the diet this is no longer true) that it can't be a diet that is naturally good for you. For a long time I just accepted this as a fact of life, an imperfection in an otherwise perfect dietary solution. But the story of B12 is much bigger than that.

The ultimate source of B12 is a bacteria found in soil. In fact, the animal sources of B12 are most commonly from soil and bacterial contamination during slaughter. Eww! It isn't something that is "naturally" in the muscle tissue of animals that they benevolently pass on to us humans. In fact, before our society became so sterile and germaphobic, humans got their B12 through the soil they worked with their hands! We are so far from our agrarian roots, in most cases, that we no longer work the soil with our hands. Even if you do work with soil, in many cases the soil too has been sterilized to the point where it is no longer a viable growing medium for the bacterial sources of B12.

So you have a choice. You can get your B12 from a high calorie, cholesterol and fat laden contaminated meat source, or from miso soup (or take a B12 vitamin).

In my mind, that's what it comes down to. Since we fight a disease that thrives on fat, we must make choices that make sense in terms of fighting obesity. We must choose to eat less of the saturated fats, not more. Do yourself a favor, eat to your advantage! Eating meat just for B12 is like saying that you need to eat an ice cream sundae so that you can get the vitamin C in the cherry.

My rule (as you know) is to err on the side of nutrition and foods that will help me fight this deadly disease. I do ask myself every day if I am eating (or drinking) the best thing I can to help my body beat (or keep beating) obesity. I have made this my practice. Choose nutrient dense foods that are very low in saturated fat, chemicals, and calories. And when in doubt, take a B Complex every day! You will thank yourself for it!

A word about antacids!

I've been known to say that over the counter anti-gas remedies are good when you begin eating more produce. It's true. But be aware that things like omeprazole (Prilosec, etc.) can rob you of magnesium and vitamin B12.

This is VITALLY IMPORTANT to those of us who fight obesity.

Magnesium works to convert blood sugar into energy. The first time I took magnesium I was struck by an amazing feeling. It was energy! Clean, unbridled energy! Not frenetic energy, the kind you get from stimulants like caffeine, but a slow clean burning energy that felt great! Magnesium also works to help calcium absorb into our bones. It's great to take them together, but I don't take a 2 in 1 product as I need more magnesium than I have seen in many of the Cal/Mag products. Just my personal preference. Besides, anything that converts blood sugar to usable energy is something I want to be sure I am getting enough of! Talk to your doctor, nutritionist or naturopath if you have questions about vitamins and your diet.

Calcium

We all know we need calcium. It is important for strong bones and teeth, and a host of other things. Nothing new there. I just wanted to mention that if you drink coffee, soda, or tea, and you don't want to lose calcium as a result, listen up. Every time I drink coffee I take calcium. Now I only drink coffee in the mornings, and most days just two cups. I'm aware that caffeine can leech calcium from our bones, so I simply compensate by taking a little extra calcium on days when I drink a bit more coffee. Calcium citrate is more bioavailable than calcium carbonate, so I take that when I take a supplement. My first recommendation for getting enough calcium, eat kale, miso or sesame seeds! Sesame seeds have more calcium than any other food source in the world!! 'Nuff Said.

Partially Hydrogenated ANYTHING

In case you missed the memo, any label that has "partially hydrogenated" or "hydrogenated" on it is something you should never put in your mouth! This process turns ordinary fats into trans fats. Trans fats are deadly. Animals do not normally have high cholesterol. When researchers want to raise the cholesterol of unwitting animal subjects, they feed them trans fats. It's the fastest, most effective way to raise your cholesterol and your risk of heart disease.

I say over and over in this book that you must listen to your body. You know your co-morbidities. You also know that if you don't have co-morbid conditions, your family history will give you a clue as to what you are most susceptible to. If your mother or father have diabetes or heart disease, it is a good bet that if you follow in their cultural footsteps, you will end up with the same diseases.

By cultural footsteps I mean that you live the same way they live. You eat roughly the same foods, prepared the same ways. You exercise in the same patterns that they do. If you handle your emotions in the same manner that they do, you are following in their cultural footsteps. For many families buying food is one of two things. It is either cheap or it is nutritious. Unfortunately, those hit hardest by other cultural issues like lack of education and economic hardships get a double whammy in this regard. Even if you want to eat healthily, the cheapest stuff in the grocery store is historically the least nutritious.

The exception to this rule is fresh produce. Often fresh produce, especially during a sale, is one of the cheapest items in the store! For the same price as a bag of potato chips you can get a pound of apples, sometimes two or three pounds. That's a deal when you think about how satisfying apples are compared with chips. Chips and other processed snacks are empty calories. I've heard that term my whole life and I understand it better now than I ever have. Empty calories are not satisfying. The important bit to recognize here is that food ads are designed to convince you that their candy bar or bag of chips is as satisfying as sex. Literally. And we watch them so many times without any thought for their purpose and the fact that they are lying to us. We simply accept that the wonderful warm feelings that are released when we eat this junk (much processed chocolate is in this category too by the way) are present because the food is inherently good for us.

That could not be farther from the truth. The warm fuzzy feelings we are experiencing after a candy bar are from the same source as if you just drank a mild radioactive solution. YES! Endorphins rush into your blood stream to calm you and make you feel good in a self defense move, because you have just done something that has CAUSED YOU BODILY HARM! Endorphins are hormones that are natural pain killers. If you eat bad food-like substances, very often you will experience endorphins in order to counteract the pain you are causing yourself. In fact, the body is so good at this that you never even experience it as pain. It just registers in your brain as pleasure. Make no mistake, food scientists have known this for decades.

One of the problems with this (and there are many) is that eventually your endorphins will stop working as effectively as they should. What that means is that in an accident you might be counting on endorphins to get you through the extreme pain, and they won't work as well as if you had not abused them for years. Many researchers believe that this is one reason that obesity is so physically painful. Besides issues like the obvious natural joint erosion due to excess weight, obesity makes us susceptible to experiencing more pain at lower thresholds (Guneli, Gumustekin, Ates, 2010). What's interesting about this is that the research points to a link between a hormone called ghrelin that tells us that we are hungry. In people without obesity, eating lowers the amount of ghrelin in your body. That shuts off the hunger sensation. In addition, researchers think that this failure to lower the amount of ghrelin in our system also makes us susceptible to pain at lower thresholds. So, you and I experience pain long before our healthier counterparts possibly because we have too much ghrelin in our bodies.

This is a complex issue. No doubt. Suffice it to say, eat things that do not cause your body pain. You wouldn't drink radioactive water. Don't eat food-like substances. Be able to identify the exact foods you are eating; every single ingredient. Just because the package calls them blueberry muffins, doesn't mean there are any blueberries in them. While blueberries are very good for you, manufactured blueberry-like muffins cause you pain, in so many ways!

Write Your Story

Is there a food, or a specific meal that you associate with something pleasant from your childhood?

Do you use that food for comfort now? Why or why not?

MAGIC MUSHROOMS

Groovy Baby!
Mushrooms are about the closest thing to magic that I am aware of. Maybe not in the way you might be thinking right now, but they are simply amazing and I propose that in order to fight obesity we cannot afford to live without them. Mushrooms are about the closest thing to magic that I am aware of. Maybe not in the way you might be thinking right now, but they are simply amazing and I propose that in order to fight obesity we cannot afford to live without them.

First I should tell you what phytochemicals are. Phytochemicals or phytonutrients are simply beneficial chemicals that come from plants. We have known for years now that oats can help lower cholesterol. That's great, but it is small in comparison to what mushrooms, onions, pomegranates, and greens can do!

The Mushroom Miracle
Ok, maybe it's not a Vatican-verified miracle, but pretty darn amazing! Mushrooms are so important to fighting obesity, and such an unsung hero in the fight that I had to give them a chapter of their own!

I can hear the American groans now. So many people dislike mushrooms that this may constitute a true challenge. Despite how you feel about mushrooms now, when you find out how important they are, you will probably want to find a way to work them into your diet!

Mushrooms are a centuries old, very effective home remedy that have been used to aid in fighting inflammation, lowering blood pressure, blood sugar, cholesterol, and are also effective in fighting and preventing the growth of many forms of cancer. On top of all that they help in the fight against bacterial and viral infections! WHAT? YES! Mushrooms have a good amount of protein, iron, riboflavin and niacin and they are high in fiber too! Still most Americans do not eat a wide variety of mushrooms with any regularity. When was the last time you ate mushrooms? I think the key is in understanding and preparation. We'll get to that later!

The amazing nutrient value of mushrooms is wonderful, but for the purposes of fighting the battle we wage against excess fat, mushrooms are uniquely powerful!

First, mushrooms are a well known fat burning food. While you are enjoying them for their nutrients and flavors, they are burning fat for you! This is amazing to me! Why aren't we eating these more often!?

Mushrooms are useful in our fight against fat in that they promote fat metabolism and work to restrict the growth of fat cells!!!! It is true (Fuhrman, 2012; Kohno, Miyake, Sano, et al., 2008; Borchers, Keen, Gershwin, 2004; Martin & Brophy, 2010).

They also improve digestion and help you feel satisfied after eating! Many studies have shown mushroom's power to metabolize fat and prevent weight regain! Here's how!

Here Come the Juicy Bits!

The most significant way mushrooms aid in weight loss and prevent weight regain is by a process that interferes with something called angiogenesis. Angiogenesis is the development of new blood vessels in the body. You might think at first blush that angiogenesis is a good thing. It is in childhood and during pregnancy! But the problems come with excess angiogenesis in adulthood. Why are these blood vessels so important? Because it is through blood that nutrients and oxygen are carried to the various parts of our bodies. Think about a cancerous tumor. Abnormal cells, cancer, and fat cells all produce angiogenesis promoting compounds that are designed to keep them alive and growing! Once the tumor is large enough the body begins to build blood cells to support the tumor and keep it alive. In the same way, when fatty areas on the body become large enough angiogenesis kicks in and we form blood vessels to support the fat, keep it alive and help it to continue to expand! Think about that! Without eating even one more calorie, fat has its own built in growth mechanism! This was handy for survival during famines but really backfires in a culture with too much food. Is it any wonder that it is difficult to lose weight and keep it off?

You have undoubtedly heard in the news that there is a connection between obesity and certain cancers. This is at least one of those connections! Fat and cancer both promote, with the help of an unhealthy diet, angiogenesis. The biggest culprits in producing angiogenesis are white flour, high sugar, high fat, and high cholesterol foods. You would do well to steer clear of those things! They actually encourage and support fat expansion!

Mushrooms also contain Antigen-binding lectins (ABL), are proteins that bind only to abnormal cells. This is cool because once they have bound themselves to the cell they interfere with its ability to continue to grow out of control (Yu, Fernig, Smith, et al., 1993).

Anti-aromatase compounds actually reduce the estrogen levels in women, which in turn lowers the risk that estrogen will cause cancer to grow. Mushrooms also contain these important anti-aromatase compounds. Mushrooms that are high in protective anti-aromatase compounds include the white button, white stuffing, cremini, portobello, reishi, and maitake. You can (and should) cook these because cooking will kill any harmful bacteria while it does not disturb the incredible health benefits!

Mushrooms are a powerful weapon in the fight against obesity.

I would go so far as to say that mushrooms are nearly as important in the diet of an obesity patient as insulin is to a diabetic patient. Think of mushrooms as a medicine that works to help cure (yes I said cure) obesity. Because mushrooms inhibit angiogenesis which slows the growth of blood vessels into fatty tissues, the theory is that fat is much more easily released from the body! If the fat isn't supported by blood, it is less likely to remain in storage. In the same way, if tumors do not maintain a blood supply, they shrink and die. If however, veins and vessels grow into our fatty areas, the body sees that fat as an important part of our bodily structure, which we then automatically strive to retain and support.

Similarly, onions are powerful against angiogenesis! Eat them together for an even bigger effect! Onions are in a food category called alliums. This group includes foods like leaks, shallots, chives, and scallions.

Pomegranates and berries are another weapon that belongs in your anti-obesity arsenal. I hear complaints all the time about how expensive good foods are for you, but this is only true for certain good foods, and it is a short term thinking problem. It is by far cheaper to buy berries and fresh mushrooms than to pay (in so many ways) for a coronary bypass or knee replacements due to osteoarthritis. Think about the $30 you spend on pizza for your family! Replace pizza and soda or eating out with mushrooms and onions and you could save a lot of money!

Pomegranates deserve their own chapter as far as health producing benefits! According to recent research, pomegranate seeds (and the juice too) lower blood pressure, lower your risk of cancer and heart disease, build bone density in animal tests, reverses atherosclerosis by 30%, and improve the symptoms of depression!* If you are really smart you would have a salad every day at lunchtime with all these things in it!!

So, you want to shed excess fat? Use these foods as weapons against it! See a more complete list in Chapter 11.

So, to release the stored fat, and to keep it off, eat mushrooms every single day!! I have started a practice of eating cooked mushrooms and onions between 2 and 3pm daily. This is my "danger time zone". You know what I am referring to. It's the time of day when you are most likely to eat something that isn't good for you. Maybe your energy flags during a different time of day. Maybe mid morning and mid afternoon you tend to grab a snack. It is not uncommon. I fry up a 3 day batch of mushrooms and onions (I like red onions personally) in an olive oil spray until the onions are caramelized and the mushrooms are well cooked. Each day I reheat the mushrooms before eating them, which by the way does not take away from the medicinal effects! It is important to cook mushrooms as some research indicates that certain types of uncooked mushrooms can be dangerous. That's a precaution, not something that should stop you from eating them.

Some of the best mushrooms are shiitake, maitake, enokitake, porcini, ink cap, portobello, champignon, crimini, and pioppino. Even the common white button variety has this important effect and is also high in B vitamins which contributes to better moods! And you don't have to eat a cup of mushrooms at a time to get this effect.

In fact, eating one medium sized white button mushroom a day can decrease your cancer risk by up to 89%! It's that powerful!

If you suffer, as I do, from autoimmune diseases mushrooms are essential. Many of them have immuno-regulatory functions! So many people in highly developed Western nations have in recent years developed environmental allergies, RA and a host of other autoimmune diseases. This is a result of our autoimmune systems running amok! In Eastern cultures (like China and Japan) that include a lot of these mushrooms in their diet you see a lot less obesity and autoimmune problems. It might be that mushrooms are far more important than we ever thought possible!

Another important nutrient in many types of mushrooms is Vitamin D. Having just moved to Washington state I find it interesting that in a place where the sun doesn't shine a lot, mushrooms grow prolifically. It is wonderful how nature has provided a readily available source of Vitamin D in a place where the sun doesn't shine enough to provide it.

Today many of us regardless of climate simply do not get enough sunlight to have therapeutic amounts of vitamin D in our bodies. You can take a daily walk and you can also count on mushrooms to help you with getting enough Vitamin D! Taking a walk has a whole lot of other benefits. So, hedge your bets. Do both!

An Acquired Taste

Just for your general information, everything edible is actually an acquired taste. EVERYTHING! You can condition yourself to like (or dislike) any food. When you were a kid you may have turned your nose up at broccoli, but as an adult it may have become one of your favorite veggies. How did that happen?

It takes, according to some researchers, just three instances of eating a certain kind of food before you begin to like it. Just three. Some things don't take even three times, like sweet or salty foods for example. You may like those right away. But for things that are foreign or unusual in your diet, three is the magic number. Some foods, like mushrooms and kale, are worth the effort of acquiring a taste for them. Anything that jam packed with nutrients and fat busting properties is worth it! And if you just can't get there, check with your neighborhood herbalist, naturopath or health food store. They may have them in pill form. My preference is always to get nutrients through whole foods, but these nutrients are too important to miss out on just because you don't like them.

Another great option is to chop or grind mushrooms into tiny bits and substitute half mushrooms and half ground meat (rather than all meat) in hot dishes, meat balls, tacos and other combination meals. I do not recommend meat, especially red meat. But if you are bent on eating it, do yourself a favor and add mushrooms.

PAY ATTENTION

Beginnings are fun. Everything is new and exciting and there is change everywhere. This is especially true for diet and exercise programs. That's why we buy so many diet books! It's exciting! When we first begin a new program we are excited at the prospect of what that program can do for us. We put our best foot forward and things look pretty good! Unfortunately before too long, the other shoe drops and we are back to square one. As a society, we are really good at beginnings. This is part of why so many diets appear to work in the first weeks but don't last. The problem is very simple, but important none-the-less. In the beginning of a new diet you are very strict, you pay attention to every detail as if your life depends upon it. You pour all kinds of energy and time into the details of the new diet, and you hold your own feet to the fire... in the beginning.

Paying attention is the thing that gradually goes away as we become more confident in the diet rules. Before too long we stop measuring our food; after all it is a big hassle and nearly impossible when you eat out. And then your nephew's birthday comes up and you rationalize that a tiny bite or two of cake won't make much of a difference.... until it does. Then there is an office celebration and you worked so hard! And life just starts to get into the way of the strict diet rules. After all, you have to live, right? And it's not like your life depends upon this particular diet.

The thing to understand is that your life literally does depend upon you managing this disease. Not just your life, which many people cannot really grasp in this context, but your quality of life. Is there anyone on earth who feels better when they have morbid obesity than when they don't? If there is, I assure you the pleasure will be short lived. As your body ages you go through all kinds of changes that weaken you over time. There's nothing (yet) that we can do about this. If you are healthy and fit those changes are manageable. If you have a disease those changes can come more quickly and they are a lot tougher to manage. Your veins, your bones, your organs all suffer under the pressure of obesity. They also suffer as you age. Obesity as you age is a double whammy! That's why there are so few 400 pound 90 year olds! I'm not actually sure it has happened yet!

Quality of life encompasses a whole range of things, including how you are treated by society.

The research is clear on this. People who suffer from obesity are more likely to be thought of as lazy, incompetent, and less intelligent. That's not my idea of fun. Whether or not you put stock in what others think, it affects you. It affects the amount of money you can earn. It affects the people you date and ultimately mate with. It affects your own self respect, if you are honest. It affects how long you have to live and whether or not you will see your daughter married, or even your grandchildren grown and married.

The point here is that it is in your long term best interest in so many ways to manage your disease diligently. Not just for a few weeks, or until you lose weight. Remember, weight loss is not the cure for obesity. It is simply the removal of one symptom. If you do not continue to pay attention, no matter what you choose to do about diet and exercise, you will fail. I promise you.

If you have high blood pressure, for example, and you choose not to pay attention to it, it is likely to continue to get higher. If you have diabetes and fail to pay attention to it you will die. The same holds true for obesity.

So when you begin a new program and start to make changes and experience success, enjoy it! But this time make at point to continue to pay attention for the long haul.

There are gurus out there who theorize about how you should change your eating and diet patterns periodically. The rules are complex and sometimes ridiculous! Eat carbs one day, then no carbs, then limit calories for two days before you take a day off to binge. They won't usually tell you that what's working is that you are simply paying attention. Some of them don't even know that's why their programs work in the short term. I contend that is exhausting and unsustainable in the very long term. But I will agree that they are onto something. It does cause you to pay close attention to what you eat. That's the important part. If you can simply pay attention you don't have to put yourself through all the rest of it!

Look, it sucks to have to pay attention to what you eat and to make sure you are moving enough. There are some people who are thin who seem oblivious to how they eat and they never exercise, yet they are tiny! First of all, they probably don't have the disease called obesity. Secondly, they might have better genes than you were saddled with. Nothing you can do about that yet either! Thirdly, you probably have no idea what their habits really are from day to day. Many people are very different in private than their public persona would suggest. Lastly, when I first began to jog avidly it struck me that nearly all of my thin friends were runners or what I called "secret athletes". I had no idea before I began running that any of them participated in anything remotely athletic. I was stunned that I had no idea about these activities and how prevalent it was among my healthy friends. You might be assuming that they are as sedentary as you are! We tend to judge others by our own experiences. It just never dawned on me that they were that much more active than I was. Maybe you are much more self aware than I was. Maybe something in your head has allowed you to push notions of being active off as something that just "wasn't you".

One last point. Consistency is foundational. It takes true courage to be consistent. It takes strength and tenacity. Consistency masquerades as boring and unimaginative; less than spontaneous. Spontaneity gets all the attention, after all! From the outside it looks fun and unpredictable and creative. But it takes a lot more creativity and imagination to be consistent for the long term than it does to be spontaneous. Spontaneity is just compulsivity disguised as fun. It plays to our weakness and feeds discontent.

"It's not what we do once in a while that shapes our lives. It's what we do consistently."

— Anthony Robbins

Tony Robbins is spot on. If your life is spontaneous you will never get anywhere. We see all these movies and books where being spontaneous is the answer to all the problems afflicting our main character. The problem is that we forget that the reason it is the "answer" is that the person has been consistently "plodding along" in their lives to the exclusion of any kind of fun. That's not what consistency offers! It is just a Hollywood aberration. It is very similar to the differences between Hollywood romance and the real deal. There are nearly no similarities, save one: the beginning. In the beginning of our romances we are swept up in the exciting new relationship, nearly blind to every day life. As I said, we are really good at beginnings and it is because we have gotten a ton of training from movies, books, TV and other entertainment!

Think about it: a movie about being consistently healthy where little goes wrong wouldn't be a good movie at all. But we aren't living a movie. We are living a real life. Isn't that exactly what we want? A life that minimizes things that could go wrong? We see in the movies and TV that consistency and a well managed life are portrayed as plodding and boring and colorless. Nothing could be further from the truth! Living a consistent life means that there is time to do the fun stuff you want to do! Without consistency we can't be spontaneous! We simply would not have the resources or energy! It is the consistently managed life that is full and exciting! Rampant spontaneity is all about being compulsive and compulsivity is at the heart of obesity. Think about what it means to be spontaneous. It almost always involves eating or doing something you know isn't good for you. Once in a while it is exciting. A steady "diet" of spontaneity is not exciting and it is not healthy. It's like living on Jelly Beans! Grow up and eat your greens.

I want to challenge you to start thinking of consistent activity and paying attention to diet as essential parts of your life going forward. Create a checks and balances routine for yourself. Every two weeks, take stock of what you are doing that is working and what is not. Keep a journal. It takes just a few minutes daily to make an entry that you can use to maximize your efforts. Monthly monitor your practices, making sure that you haven't started doing anything consistently that could encourage obesity or that discourages movement. Maybe during Halloween someone put out a candy dish at their desk that you can't resist every time you walk by. What kinds of things have stopped you this month from successfully completing your health goals?

If you keep a journal, add to it a column for hunger. Get to know hunger and what real hunger feels like. When you experience hunger (real hunger) make a note of it. How long were you hungry before you ate? What did it make you think? Where you obsessed with food? Why is this important?

First of all, the physical feeling you have when you are truly hungry is the feeling of weight loss. If you do not overcompensate for it you will be losing weight! The problem is that we often overcompensate for it, especially if it goes on for very long. It's a built in reaction that we are all too familiar with. Secondly, when you pay attention to this feeling and wait for it each time before you eat, you will be more mindful and you will reinforce your weight loss and maintenance goals.

ANTI-OBESITY FOODS

As I mentioned earlier, we are in the fight of our lives. Whether you realize that or not, it is true. Literally. Food can be your enemy, or your ally. The choices you make everyday reveal which it is. Choose fast food for lunch, food is working against you. Choose super anti-obesity foods and suddenly food is your most powerful ally. And we can use all the help we can get in this fight! There are super foods, and then there are super anti-obesity foods. We have an amazing opportunity to eat strategically, thanks to modern science. But before you read about all these amazingly powerful tools, I want to mention something really important.

One look around the shelves of your local grocery store or drug store and you will see a wide array of pills that are condensed versions of chemicals "harvested" from super foods. And there are doctors endorsing them on TV weekly. Green tea extract, raspberry keytones, green coffee bean extract, and a whole array of other products have been concentrated and put into pill form to make it easier to get a lot of a certain compound into your diet. While it might be tempting to buy these potions, remember that when they create these they are taking the whole food apart, separating what appears to be a breakthrough chemical from the rest of the food. What's wrong with that? Everything! They did that with beta carotene and we ended up with people taking tons of beta carotene that was separated from the rest of the carotenes and other nutrients and as a result they increased their risk for cancer many times over (Fuhrman, 2012). It is not nice to fool with Mother Nature!

Please do not buy pills with these isolated chemicals in them. EAT THE WHOLE FOOD! When possible, eat them raw. These foods are a gift from nature that should be at the core of your menu plans in place of cheese, red meat and refined carbohydrates. They will make weight loss and long term maintenance a lot easier. In addition I want to remind you of days gone by when every evening meal used to begin with a salad. Do you remember that? I do! In more formal societies they used to call it the salad course. I grew up poor in the back woods of Northern Minnesota, and we ate a salad with almost every dinner. It had it's own plate, and we generally ate it before the main course. Somewhere along the line with the advent of TV dinners, canned veggies, and a zillion ways to make potatoes and rice, we lost the salad course. After reading this chapter, you may be inspired to bring it back!

Mushrooms have been mentioned in great detail in chapter 9, but there are several more really important foods that you might want to add to your shopping list.

Most of these foods are commonly found in grocery stores. Some may necessitate a trip to your local natural food store but I promise you the trip will be worth while! Notice there are no pre-prepared foods, shakes, or supplements on this list. All these foods are relatively low in calories, some of them nearly calorie free! Most of these things are relatively inexpensive too!

Much has been said lately about juicing. I'm not opposed to juicing if you have a problem absorbing nutrients. Most of us do not have that problem. But juicing is just another way to concentrate our food, many times adding more sugar than we need (in the form of fruit to mask the taste of the veggies) and increasing calories, breaking down enzymes, and decreasing fiber unnecessarily. Eat whole unprocessed plant based foods whenever possible. It is that simple!

There are all kinds of foods out there that are really good for you! Avocado, coconut, and a whole host of others that are generally good for you, but aren't as good for fighting obesity. This chapter is limited to foods that help wage the war against obesity and directly related maladies.

Weapons Against Obesity:

A mix of Mushrooms, onions, bell peppers, ginger and garlic, can help reduce the blood flow to fat deposits and allow you to lose weight and keep it off far more easily. I lightly fry them in an olive oil spray. I could probably write a book on the available information on mushrooms. See the mushroom chapter (9) for the scoop. Piceatannol, found in peanuts, grape seeds and skins, blueberries and passion fruit, has some amazing benefits for those of us who fight obesity. Fat cells go through a maturation process, and introducing piceatannol to your diet can actually stop that maturation process. So baby fat cells do not become mature fat deposits. Imagine what a fruit salad of grapes, blueberries, passion fruit, sprinkled with peanuts can do for you! Make it a practice to eat these daily. I love incorporating these foods into my diet especially during my high stress times or during those hours when I start feeling peckish during the afternoon.

Pomegranates are as important as mushrooms in fighting obesity. They promote the same kind of reduction in blood flow to fat deposits. I'm not sure I can emphasize how amazing this discovery is in the fight against obesity!! Every day I eat either pomegranates or mushrooms or sometimes both. Every single day. Berries have similar properties.

Apples and Pears are very high in fiber and are natural diuretics so if you carry a lot of extra water weight you may want to eat at least one apple a day. Studies show that people who eat 3 apples or pears a day are more likely to lose weight than people who do not eat apples or pears daily. In addition to that apples (Green Tea and dark chocolate) contain an amazing substance called catechins that scientists are saying may have a protective effect on the brain after a stroke. It's also being studied for its effect on allergies. If you eat foods high in catechins, it is possible it will reduce your body's tendency to produce histamine which is what makes you miserable during allergy season. Studies are showing interesting and hopeful effects of catechins on Alzheimer's and Parkinson's diseases too. Açaí oil is high in catechins, as are peaches and vinegar. Açaí is one of the highest anti-oxidant foods on the planet.

Kale is an important calcium source, and as with all cruciferous greens is a staple in the fight against obesity and incidentally, heart disease and cancer too. Cruciferous greens include cabbage, brussels sprouts, broccoli, bok choy, cauliflower, rutabaga, turnip greens and a whole lot more!

Celery was identified as a cure for pain as far back as 30 AD and it contains a chemical called 3-n-butylphthalide which has been shown in some studies to lower blood pressure in rats. Another great thing about celery is that it has very few calories and is rich in fiber. Both great weight loss properties. If you are someone who just feels the need to crunch or chew a lot, you might want to keep celery on hand. If after your meal you still want to chew, eat ice chips or celery rather than a second helping or dessert. The rumors of celery being a negative calorie food are most likely apocryphal.

Black sesame seeds are wondrous! I keep them by the salt and pepper shakers and sprinkle them on just about everything I eat. They contain more calcium than any other food available. They boast a very high level of natural antioxidants and are very high in protein. They contain phytosterols that are associated with lowering cholesterol and regulating hormone fluctuations. When you grind regular sesame seeds you get a paste called tahini, which is a standard ingredient in humus. While humus is generally pretty expensive in the store, it can be made at home for a small fraction of the price! It is easy and when you make it at home you can choose to add any flavors that appeal to you like bell peppers, spinach, jalapeños, red onion, Italian spices, or just about any savory flavor you can think of! I love humus with celery! Two super foods in one meal!

Seeds are really important in terms of health and vitality. Think of them as itty bitty powerhouses. They are the food equivalent of stem cells, in terms of their power to heal and nourish us. Pumpkin seeds and Flax seeds are packed with Omega 3s as well as zinc, calcium and iron! Seeds are high in protein, filling and highly protective.

Phytochemicals in freshly harvested plant foods may be destroyed or removed by modern processing techniques, including cooking. In other words, cooked and highly processed foods are simply not as good for you. This is especially true of greens. And adding ham hocks to cooked greens... yeah, no longer a health food.

Quercetin is a plant derived substance found in fruits, vegetables, leafy greens and grains. It is important in fighting depression. Since depression has been correlated with obesity in many studies, it is important that we do whatever we can to fight both diseases as naturally as possible. One good way to do both is by eating more fruits and veggies. One great choice is watermelon. It's high in lycopene and beta carotene and preliminary research indicates the consumption of watermelon may lower blood pressure.

Oxalic Acid which we get in both spinach and green tea has been shown to inhibit tumor growth. This is important because obesity has been linked to several different cancers. Phthalides which are found in celery is reported to lower blood pressure. Celery also has antioxidants, fiber and is a natural anti-inflammatory.

Spirulina has been described as one of the world's most miraculous foods. It has high quantities of vitamins B1 (thiamine), B2 (riboflavin), B3 (nicotinamide), B6 (pyridoxine), B9 (folic acid), vitamin C, vitamin D, vitamin A and vitamin E. It is also a source of potassium, calcium, chromium, copper, iron, magnesium, manganese, phosphorus, selenium, sodium and zinc. Sounds like a multivitamin doesn't it!

Miso Soup is a wonder food too! I have begun a practice in which I eat it nearly every morning for breakfast as they do in Japan. Miso soup helps balance your intestinal tract and helps you to digest, synthesize, and absorb nutrients. The more nutrients that you can effectively digest means fewer cravings, and a lower satiation threshold. By strengthening your intestinal fortitude this incredible soup strengthens your immune system and helps you fight off sickness. From NaturalNews.com: "Benefits include reduced risks of breast, lung, prostate, and colon cancer, and protection from radiation. Researchers have found that consuming one bowl of miso soup per day, as do most residents of Japan, can drastically lower the risks of breast cancer."

Anti-inflammatory Foods:

Some of the most important anti-inflammatory vegetables are broccoli, cabbage, garlic, spinach, leeks, green beans, Brussels sprouts, bok choy, and spring onions. Fish is a wonderfully anti-inflammatory food, especially salmon and other varieties that are high in Omega 3 oils. However please understand the risks both to you and the environment when you eat certain kinds of fish or seafood. A great reference for this is The Environmental Defense Fund. You can find them at http://apps.edf.org/page.cfm?tagID=1521 Before I found this site I thought our locally caught (Washington state) salmon, for example, was perfectly safe to eat. Turns out that recommendations for adults include eating it just once a month because of PCBs found in it. Children should eat only half a serving a month. Be careful and know the facts. It is also good to know where your fish comes from. If you don't know, ask your grocer or the folks who sell you the fish.

Chili peppers which contain a metabolism boosting substance called capsaicin, which is also anti-inflammatory and reportedly a pain killer. Triple bonus!

I cannot emphasize enough the importance of beneficial omega 3 oils. Foods that contain this life enhancing nutrient include salmon and other cold fresh water fish like and herring, tuna, and sardines. Other sources include olives, nuts, seeds, kale, spinach, flax seeds, walnuts, soybeans, and broccoli. I am sensing a trend here! Incorporate them into your menu plans! A lack of dietary Omega 3 is linked to depression and anxiety and a whole host of mental illnesses. It is also linked to inflammation, heart disease, dry, itchy, or flakey skin, fatigue and poor circulation. Omega 3 is pretty important! Use food to your benefit!

One word about eggs. Some eggs are "engineered" to be higher in omega 3. Chickens who are fed flax seeds produce eggs with high levels of Omega 3 oil. This sounds good on the surface, but it lacks a holistic approach. Think about the fact that eggs also contain high levels of cholesterol. I can't prove it now, but I think research down the road will find issues with omega 3 enriched eggs. I have other problems with eggs, based on industrial practices. But we will see in time how history and science judge these eggs and if they really are as good for us as some say. For now, I'm sticking to plant and fish based omega 3 sources that have always had it, without our intervention. What's important here is that you find out what works for you! If eggs work for you, and your blood tests, weight, mood, etc. all concur, eat them! There is no one thing that works for everyone. Eggs have no carbs, so for someone with diabetes, they might be a good protein source. For others who worry about heart disease, eggs may not be the best food choice.

Think about what you are practicing.

If you eat eggs every morning, you have made a practice of it. Be mindful in your practices, make choices, especially around those things you do every single day, that give you your best fighting chance at beating obesity and poor health.

This is by no means a complete list of super foods. The list is growing all the time thanks to food scientists. And these amazing foods have more nutrients than are possible to mention in these pages. But this is a good place to start.

Make as many of these a part of your daily diet as possible. They vary in price and availability of course but these days we have much of this available to us year round. You can always get greens and generally speaking, they are very inexpensive. I recommend kale and spinach daily. Maybe just add a green salad before your main course at dinner. See the Raw Kale Recipe box to get in on the amazing secret that made kale more enjoyable and accessible for me and my family.

Please note: There is no legal definition of the term "Superfood". It is a marketing term that was created to get at the idea that certain foods have very high nutrient content. One of the more benign marketing terms out there. However, like a lot of what I am telling you - simplicity is the key. Does a food possess a high level of plant nutrients? That's another word that gets used a lot that sounds way more mysterious than it really is: Phytonutrients. It means plant nutrients. That's it.

Another Note: Although this book isn't a diet book, it is a book about a disease that is affected by diet and exercise. It is for that reason that I am including the information about food and eating habits, as well as what real exercise is. They are not by any means mandates or some kind of diet craze. They are simple, common sense things to consider that may help you manage this disease. Think of this food list as the most helpful tool in your arsenal as you fight obesity and return to vitality!

Write Your Story

Keep a food diary for a week. Keep times and food choices logged.

What do you do consistently? Do you drink coffee daily? What time of day do you drink coffee? How does it make you feel (physically and emotionally)? Do you eat oatmeal every morning?

When the week is finished, look at your daily habits to discover your practices.

What are you practicing? Are you practicing chips in front of the TV every night? Do you eat a snack before bed every night?

When is your "weakest" part of the day when you make the worst choices? The only way to be mindful of your practices is to study them!

Now that you have found what you practice think about how you could change your practices to reinforce good healthy practices. Use those daily habits to fight obesity rather than to encourage it. If you have a snack before bed, maybe eating a small salad or a handful of seeds would be a better choice than ice cream or something else. Find out what works for you.

Start a new healthy practice this week.

MOVE!

It is amazing to me that we who live in developed nations can have so much available to us in terms of resources and education and we are still some of the fattest, most unhealthy people in the world! Of course these advantages are a double edged sword. With great gifts come great responsibilities. And it is certainly easy to overindulge when food is so plentiful.

In most large cities there are gyms aplenty. Even small towns have workout facilities now. Heck, the great outdoors is there for the taking! And it is free! But even if we are motivated to purchase a membership we don't use them. It is true that home exercise equipment is used more as a makeshift closet than for exercise.

Point is, we don't move. I've said it before, and I will continue to say it: You cannot be healthy if you do not move! If you want to be healthy, you must find a way to move every day. That's all there is to it.

The reality for many people who struggle with obesity is that movement is so painful that you just can't do it with any regularity. This is especially true for people who have co-morbidities like I do.

My pain levels are so high that I see a pain doctor at least once a month and very often even more than that. My RA and fibromyalgia prohibit me from a lot of vigorous exercises. This has been a terrible problem for me in my fight against obesity. On good days I can walk, and some weeks I can walk nearly every day. But consistency is the key, and pain flares really gum up the works. It seems just about the time I get a really consistent pattern of exercises going the pain flares up and I am back in bed! It is Very Frustrating!

I know that I am not alone in this! I have talked to countless people who suffer from co-morbidities who have the same experience with exercise. Doing light exercise, for example, can help Fibromyalgia. Unfortunately, there is a fine line to walk for folks with fibromyalgia. Too much exercise can cause a pain flare that can last for days or weeks. Too little exercise can also cause a pain flare. Inconsistent exercise can cause a flare. And experimentation to find the right balance is very often really painful and can take months. We really know so little about fibromyalgia that it is difficult for doctors to give any kind of concrete guidance. Each person's experience with it is so different, in terms of how the body responds to movement.

Fortunately, we do know a few things about it. First, we know now that it is an autoimmune problem, and it is nerve related. Medications have been developed to help with the pain, and for many people they do. Unfortunately, the problem of obesity still plagues many people with fibromyalgia because of those medications and because of their inability to exercise consistently.

I think that I have found at least a partial solution. Isometric Exercises. It is at least a good place to begin that does no harm to joints and can really help to build muscle without any kind of jarring or impact problems. Further, it doesn't seem to bother my fibromyalgia like movement can. There is value in all kinds of movement. This particular chapter is just a primer on how to get started. But my friend, Micki reminded me of an old saying that is wonderful, "Never sit when you can stand. Never stand when you can walk. Never walk when you can run." I want to add one to that, "Never take the elevator when you can take the stairs." All movement is valuable. Make good choices that work for you every single day but be mindful of your realities.

Once you are in a position to move, and you begin a walking program or some other kind of movement program, remember the first rule of exercise. It's not exercise if you are not literally dripping sweat. My rule is that I try to do 20-30 minutes once I've have begun to drip sweat, each and every day. That means that your warm up doesn't count until you are actually dripping sweat. And your cool down doesn't count because it is likely you will continue to drip sweat for a while after you stop exercising. Be true to yourself. Do the time, and do it right. Move until you are dripping. Then move for another 20-30 minutes. It may take you 20 minutes to get to the point of dripping, if you are in good physical condition. It may be that walking out your front door starts the sweat pouring down your face. That's ok, just move.

In my current condition, I walk for about half a mile or so before I begin to drip sweat. I'm not in very good condition. And it is common for some morbidly obese people to sweat all the time. For others it doesn't take much to break a sweat. I'm not talking about beads of sweat on your forehead; I'm talking and sweat streaming down your face, getting into your eyes, forcing you to wipe it off. This is important because this is one of the avenues through which your body discards fat. Sweat and urine are the two ways you lose fat. If you want to lose fat you must sweat and or pee it out. That's all there is to it. So, drink a lot of water, and move until you are dripping sweat.

So how much water is enough? The Institute of Medicine determined that an adequate intake (AI) for men is roughly 3 liters (about 13 cups) of total beverages a day. The AI for women is 2.2 liters (about 9 cups) of total beverages a day (MayoClinic.com, 2012). That's pretty close to the famed 8 - 8 oz. glasses a day. But remember, you have a disease. This disease changes what is considered adequate for your body. If you are carrying more weight, you must drink more.

My bariatric surgeon told me once that in addition to the 8 - 8 ounce glasses, each day I should drink 8 ounces of water for every 10 pounds of excess weight I was carrying. That's a lot of water for some people. Do the math! If you are carrying an extra 40 pounds of weight that's 64 oz. (baseline) plus 4 more 8 ounce glasses of water a day! That's 96 ounces of water a day! Oh, one more thing! For every cup of coffee or soda with caffeine you drink, add another 8 ounces of water to off-set the dehydrating effects. If you drink decaf coffee, add 4 ounces for every cup.

This is important, not just for weight loss, but for the smooth functioning of your organs. If you carry excess weight it taxes your body. Every part of your body has to work harder just to live. To help your organs to work more easily, your joints to move more smoothly, drink water. In addition to helping you lose fat, water will also help you lose excess water weight. Drink water. Your kidneys will thank you!

Like many of you my typical day begins early and with coffee (not decaf) and I usually drink 2-3 cups! That's another 2-3 eight oz. glasses of water! Yikes! We're up to a whopping 96 oz. before I calculate the excess weight! Wow.

For example, if you have 80 pounds of excess weight and you drink 4 cups of regular coffee every morning, you are looking at 64 (baseline) plus 32 (the price for drinking coffee) plus another 64 (to compensate for 80 extra pounds). That brings us to 160 ounces of water a day. Think about what that means for your day. In practical terms, you really want to have a lot of it done before about 4pm. If you end up drinking too much before bed you will lose sleep to pee time. I'm just sayin'. So, get your water in early in the day.

This might seem daunting at first but I have developed just one trick that can make it a lot easier. I flavor it with lemon. Choose a fruit that you can squeeze into your water and you will have just enough flavor to enhance the water but not enough to add significant calories.

I stay away from commercial flavoring mixes. Artificial sweeteners are not your friends. Even stevia, which is the latest no calorie all natural sweetener darling, can be dangerous to you if you are (like me) allergic to ragweed, daisies, or other grasses and plants. It can make your liver counts skyrocket, and it increases the acid in your body's Ph which is not a good thing. It is important to err on the side of alkalinity. I won't go into a lot on Ph levels. Suffice it to say that an acidic diet can lead to severe bone loss and a whole host of other serious issues.

From WebMD.com, "Stevia is used as a weight loss aid; for treating diabetes, high blood pressure and heartburn; for lowering uric acid levels; for preventing pregnancy; and for increasing the strength of the muscle contractions that pump blood from the heart. Not enough is known about the use of stevia during pregnancy and breast-feeding. Stay on the safe side and avoid use. Stevia might cause an allergic reaction in people who are sensitive to the Asteraceae/Compositae family of plants. This family includes ragweed, chrysanthemums, marigolds, daisies, and many other plants."

Having said all that, I do not believe that it is effective as a contraceptive, as it has not been approved for this use. I do not want to hear from people telling me that they took "my advice" and got pregnant despite using stevia! First, I do not recommend stevia. And if you use it you might want to pay attention if you are attempting to get pregnant. I do believe that it is safer than the chemically based artificial sweeteners on the market today, assuming you are not allergic to it. That's stevia in a nut shell. If you have any questions about it, please ask your doctor before you use it.

The whole point is that adding a zero calorie flavor to your water might make it easier to drink in these high volumes. My husband is fond of a bit of lemon juice in his water. It doesn't have to be sweet to be effective.

Using zero calorie sodas, even those sweetened with natural sweeteners, isn't the same as drinking water and doesn't count toward your water intake for the day. The carbonation isn't good for your bones or stomach, and much of it contains caffeine and a whole lot of other chemicals that you really don't want to ingest in large amounts. So, stay away from diet sodas in general. See my earlier warning about diet pop.

Another reason water is important is because it supports you during movement. Whenever you go out to walk, run, or get any kind of exercise you risk dehydration. This is particularly important if you live in the desert. So, add that to your water calculations. If you live in a dry, arid place where it does not rain regularly, or your area is involved in a drought, your water intake must reflect those variables. I would add at least one 8 oz. glass a day to compensate for living in those dry areas. That's not a scientific solution, just my personal preference. And you should listen to your body. Always listen to your body first.

Remember to consider the environment before you go out. Heed pollution warnings if you live in a large city. The heat or cold outside can change your need for water too. As I write this I am in the desert where, if I exercise outdoors in the summertime I am in danger of heatstroke, dehydration and all kinds of problems like kidney stones and salivary gland stones and infections of various kinds. These things can happen if I fail to drink enough water in the desert. In Minnesota, where I grew up and have spent a considerable amount of time the problem is cold. Be aware that when you do vigorous exercise your clothing must also reflect that. Dress as if the weather is 20-25 degrees warmer than it actually is. Once your body warms up and you begin to sweat, this will help you not to overheat- this is even important in the winter weather of MN. That means if it is 110 degrees F in the desert, it will feel more like 130 degrees! Use common sense. There is no way that you can prepare yourself enough to exercise in 130 degree weather. So, stay inside. On the flip side, it opens the range of weather that you might like to exercise in while in cold weather environments. It might be 25 degrees F in Minnesota, but when your body warms up it will feel more like 45 degrees. That doesn't sound too bad! Remember, 80 degrees may feel like 100 once you are moving vigorously. Use your head. If you are ambling, these rules do not apply.

Wear clothes that do not restrict your movements and choose something that wicks the moisture away from your body because even in the cold, you will sweat. I have to interject a side comment here. Various well meaning people have told me over the years that one sure way to keep the weight off is to wear restrictive clothing. They told me to never wear sweats, even at home after work. There is a nugget of truth to the awareness tight jeans bring when you begin to gain weight. However, I am not ok with being uncomfortable all day long! And the vast majority of people do not look good in tight jeans! Honestly! To that end I have started wearing tight underwear. I wear something just one size smaller than usual. But I wear my clothes to fit properly. No muffin tops here! Another idea that I got from my friend Micki (she's Gayle to my Oprah!) is to wear a snug belt. I still get the same awareness effect as I did wearing tight jeans, but now I don't have to announce it to the whole world! And don't go to extremes with this! Cutting of your circulation is not a sustainable strategy. <wry grin>

Again, listen to your body. And if the weather outside will stop you from exercising, it is better to find a way to get your exercise indoors. And in many climates that is the best way to go. I found that the desert was inhospitable for outdoor exercise on most days, with the exception of the outdoor pool. That's just based on how my body felt. I do not like the heat. So I gravitate toward indoor exercise while in hot and dry climates. But in Minnesota I loved running (prior to my RA diagnosis) in the winter weather. There were very few days I didn't run outdoors there, because I found it refreshing. Weird, I know! Even the hardy Minnesotans were looking at me askance! I know I keep saying this, but you need to think about what will work for you. What will keep you moving during the winter? or if you are in Arizona, the summer?

The common complaint is that health clubs are expensive. Costhelper.com puts the average monthly dues at a health club at between $35 and $40. Some include an initial enrollment fee, but often you can get them to waive that. If you sign a contract for six months or a year, the average monthly rate drops 25% t0 between $26 and $30 a month. Now look at what you spend on coffee or diet coke or lunch out (for example) every month. The average person who eats lunch out, rather than packing a lunch pays $37 a month for the privilege. Sixty six percent of working folks eat lunch out every day. Coffee expenses cost Americans on average $20 a week, more the younger you are. That's $1,092 a year! At $40 a month for a gym membership, you are only spending $480 a year! (http://consumerist.com). There really is no good excuse for not exercising. When the economy is slow it pays to try to negotiate with these places. You will be surprised at what you can get at a discount just for asking!

Always leave word with someone- even a note is better than nothing- when you go outside to exercise. This is particularly important in rural areas. Let someone know where you are going, what time you left and when you expect to return. That way if there is an emergency, it would be easier to find you. And I always carry a fully charged cell phone. I used it for assistance when I hurt my ankle one day and a different day when a strange man in a car kept circling each block I was running on and yelling rude comments at me, I called 911. It's easy to carry a phone, and it's a good security measure.

Bottom line: move until you drip sweat for at least 30 minutes and drink according to your weight loss requirements. And don't forget to use common sense. Always take water and a phone with you when you exercise outdoors!

I have to add something for perspective. Movement is vital to our health. I hope you hear that. But please understand that movement is not going to overcome bad eating habits. Think about it in terms of calories. If you eat a Big Mac and a super sized french fry you have eaten 1230 calories. Add another 410 for a coke and you'll have 1640 calories to burn off. That's just one meal of your day! Eat out twice in one day and you've doubled that! Now, what would you have to do to burn off just 1640 calories in a workout? Two hours of high impact aerobics and 30 minutes of racquet ball only burns 1560 calories. You would have to add another 10 minutes on the elliptical trainer to burn just over 1700 calories! That's a two hour forty minute workout daily just to compensate for a bad lunch pick! Wow! Where is that time coming from? My point is simple really. Exercise cannot compensate for bad food choices. The rule of thumb is that diet takes the weight off, exercise helps you maintain it. The reason that is true has to do with building and maintaining muscle mass. When you have more muscle mass you burn calories at a much higher rate all day long than when you have less muscle. This is the reason that those folks on the TV show "The Biggest Loser" can exercise six hours a day and still gain weight! It is so much easier to eat huge amounts of calories than it is to burn them. It takes seconds to consume what it takes hours to burn. Do yourself a big favor and when you eat something this week, measure the food in calorie burn costs, rather than just calories. So a Big Mac, fries and a coke costs you two hours and 40 minutes of your life. Count calories this way and I guarantee you will think before you eat! If you do less rigorous workouts, like playing badminton for example, that same meal will cost you well over four hours! If you swim it will cost you three hours. Do Yoga and you can count on spending four hours. You'd better start planning now if you walk for exercise! Walking that meal off will also cost you over four hours. You've got to ask yourself, even if you have that much time to spare, is it worth it? This says nothing of the content of the meal and how bad it is for your heart, liver, and other vital organs. Just start thinking about the cost before you eat.

To calculate your calorie burns you can find calculators online.

One easy to use tool is at
http://exercise.about.com/cs/fitnesstools/l/blcalorieburn.htm

Keep a calorie log that uses your particular exercise choice as a measurement of what your food will cost you.

APPROACH AVOIDANCE & THE TEMPTATIONS

Approach avoidance & the Temptations sounds like an indie band to me!

There's a phrase I just love, which has helped me through this problem more times than I want to admit. It has become a sort of mantra for me. It is: The Courage to Start. The Courage to Start is so important when it comes to exercise in particular that once you are aware of it, I hope it will change your life like it did mine.

Approach Avoidance is a type of inner conflict that happens when you must make a decision to do something that has both positive and negative effects at the same time. Like exercise, for example. You know it will feel good when you are finished, but you know that there will be effort and even pain involved during the exercise. That's why it is so difficult to get off the sofa, get your shoes on and get out the door! You are experiencing approach avoidance. Rest assured, it's common! And you don't have to have obesity for exercise to create this inner conflict! This is common for nearly all of us.

The good news is that if you are experiencing approach avoidance, you are half way there! This is evidence that you are at least thinking about exercise! There are a few things you can do to minimize the effects of the approach avoidance conflict.

One thing that I have done is that I commit to 10 minutes, no matter what. It has never failed me. Once you have your shoes on and you are out the door and you actually begin, it becomes easier to do more. Those first ten minutes are crucial. That's the warm up. By the time you have warmed up and you are headed into the dripping sweat portion of your exercise you have conquered the beast and you will be granted the strength to finish. It is amazing how well it works. It is another reason that my exercise recommendation is to literally drip sweat for 30 minutes. Rather than simply working out for a total of 30 minutes, dripping sweat before you begin counting means that you have finished the warm up and begun your workout in earnest. It's a beautifully motivating system.

Another thing that you can do is find a workout group or buddy. Having a buddy to work out with is good, but becoming part of a community that works out regularly is far better. It might be a health club class or another kind of class. I like classes framed around a goal. After my gastric bypass I began to jog and I became part of a running class at a shoe store in St. Paul, MN. That group was training for a half marathon at the time. That was a great community for me and a great goal. There are similar groups for walking and working out outdoors too. http://www.meetup.com is a great place to find free ones all over the globe. If there isn't a group you can join, start one! It's easy on meetup or you could volunteer to start one at a running/walking shoe store. I taught a "learn to run" class that was fabulous! They inspired me every single time we got together! And part of the class requirement was a 10 minute lesson each time. I think I learned more in having to teach them than any of them learned from me! You don't have to be a pro to do it and it is wonderful exercise that enriches the lives of others! Best of all you will quickly get past approach avoidance if you lead a class that's depending upon you to be there for them!

One of the easiest ways to avoid exercise is to blame the weather. If you exercise outside, which I highly recommend for many many reasons, you must have a contingency plan. By that I am not just talking about what to do when it rains or snows. I am talking about setting boundaries within which you will commit to exercise. Take into account the local climate, what's normal for your area each season. For example, in Minnesota where I grew up and have spent many years, the weather is extreme in the winter. But there are tons of folks who understand it and know how to safely dress for it and work out all winter long in Minnesota. Now, if they can do it, so can you! When we lived there I set a lower parameter of -10F degrees (real temp not including wind) that I committed to. If it was -10F or colder I did not workout outside. But anything warmer than that (I use the term 'warmer' loosely) I was out there jogging. Again, approach avoidance was tough on those cold days but I had a group of folks that I was meeting and they were waiting for me to show up before starting out. That motivation and the socialization that went with it was enough for me.

That worked for me because I am an extrovert (and I am hearty). You really need to find out what works for you. An introvert might use exercise as concentrated time alone. No outside chatter, no one needs your attention, it's just you out there doing something for you. Maybe listen to an ebook while you walk. I love that. Walk your dog! Music helps to distract me when the workout is grueling. The point is to find something that motivates you to get off the couch and do that. If you are a walker who has a big heart for the elderly you might volunteer to take some of the more active residents at an assisted living center on a walk around the area a few times a week. You may think it is beneath your fitness level, but it will enrich your life and motivate you more than you could reasonably expect. Your body will benefit too!

Hand in hand with Approach Avoidance comes Temptation. They are the evil twin sisters of unhealthy behavior. We are all familiar with Temptation. She's always there, any time your intentions are good. Any time you decide to do something that is difficult or has some kind of effort involved Temptation is there to greet you with all kinds of alternatives to the thing you know you should do. She is there when you are experiencing Approach Avoidance. She's there with her promises of comfort and ease. She's there to tell you that one day isn't enough to derail you. She's lives among the soft rules of your life.

Here's the really great news about Temptation: It turns out, she's just a bully. When I was a kid nothing scared me more than the threats of a bully. But as an adult looking at the same situation I wonder how I could have been so gullible!

Like any bully, when you stand up to Temptation she backs down. And standing up to her over and over again makes you stronger! Will power, which I think is a close opposite of Temptation, is like a muscle. The latest research tells us that we can actually strengthen the will power muscle when we use it. But it is like any other muscle. If you use it inconsistently it is not likely to get very strong. That's one of the big problems people have with will power. They don't use it daily; consistently. If you don't use it, as they say, you will lose it, like so many human experiences.

It is something you must practice. Practice is vital to everything we are talking about. If you do something regularly, in this case daily, you have made it your practice. The things you make your practice are those things that will dictate your future. It is that simple. If you do not make will power your practice you are doomed to succumb to Temptation's wiles. I like the word wiles. It means cunning behavior intended to persuade somebody to do something, especially in the form of insincere charm or flattery. That's Temptation in a nut shell, isn't it? She's not to be under estimated. But then again, neither is Will Power.

And like a bully, Temptation is insecure, weak and sad; if you look closely. Think about what Temptation is asking you to do. Temptation is asking you to join her in being weak and sad and insecure. Don't work out today, instead go to coffee and have a pastry after all it is raining outside. When you say no to Temptation you literally get stronger. When you give into her cunning behavior you literally get weaker, both in body and in mind.

Make no mistake, this is a fight. You are fighting against your habits, your years of bad choices, your old self, to establish your new identity. It's not going to happen over night. It will take time, effort, diligence, and tenacity to build the new you.

There are no tricks to building your Will Power muscles, except to make it a practice. That's the key. Use it, especially when you are truly tempted. Practice in the small things. It is powerful to overcome Temptation when it is difficult, but you will find that the more you do it, the easier it becomes. Remember too, giving into Temptation is like handing over your lunch money to the bully. That never leaves you feeling good. You've avoided your exercise, sat on the sofa through the time you are normally active. How do you feel now? Proud? Invigorated? Probably not.

Some think of it as cheating. I agree. I think you are cheating yourself out of a better quality of life. And Temptation doesn't stick around once you've given in to be your pal. She's gone and you are alone left with Guilt to console you. Not a good trade in anybody's book.

SLOW SUICIDE

I've heard obesity likened to slow suicide, but never really thought too much about it since studying psychology. Until now. I don't actually think obesity is like slow suicide, I think it is more like a half hearted suicide attempt.

We've been talking about being in this fight for our lives, and it is literal. By the same token it is by our own hand that we are here. We just don't want to admit it. The day you wake up and admit that unhealthy behaviors, especially our habits and practices, are contributing to our lowered life expectancy, is the day you really begin to fight this disease. We use all kinds of euphemisms for unhealthy eating because when it comes right down to it we would rather say we are having a "treat" than damaging our arteries. Honestly, this problem is so sensitive, so serious, and pervasive that it is difficult to approach it, even in a book about the psychological side of weight loss! But I think it is time to pull back the curtain and get real.

Seriously, I want you to know that I do not bring this up in a cavalier manner. Suicide is an issue that cuts to my heart. I lost a good friend to suicide many years ago and that is a pain that never leaves you. By the same token, this is an issue that is related to obesity and must be addressed because there are people at risk.

I have a hunch that many people who struggle long term with obesity have at least a low grade version of depression. Not everyone, but there are many people who suffer from depression who never get help. Depression is dangerous. Left untreated it can lead to suicide, and does about 80 times a day in the United States alone. Nearly one million people worldwide commit suicide each year. There are no words for how tragic this is.

It's easy to see how driving under the influence, or smoking or having unprotected sex with multiple partners might be considered reckless and self destructive. It's a lot tougher to think of that second (or third) helping of Mom's hot dish as self destructive. I remember the biggest eating trigger for me when I was a kid was when someone would say to me, "haven't you had enough yet?" or "you're getting fat! Maybe you should stop eating so much!"

Hearing that made me embarrassed and that made me angry and all I wanted to do was to eat more! Talk about a counter-productive strategy! It took a long time to get to the point where I could see over eating as my own form of self-destructive behavior. After all, I wasn't a smoker. I ate organic whole foods when ever possible. I was basically healthy if you took away the extra pounds. I certainly wasn't aware that I hated myself or that I was even depressed. But awareness is the key here. Eating because you are bored, sad, angry, need comfort, etc. is a good indication that you don't have good enough coping skills for dealing with those situations. People who cope with emotional pain with food are grasping for comfort. That could be an indication that you might be suffering from depression.

I have to interject here that in Western cultures many people view depression and in fact all psychological struggles as a socially tabooed weakness. We see these differently than we do physical or medical problems. We don't think of a broken arm as something that is taboo to talk about. Far from it! We get all our friends to support us by signing our cast and listening to our story about how we broke it! Granted, there are physical maladies that we don't talk easily about in public, but we don't judge one another for experiencing them either! (A yeast infection, for example.) And going to counseling is just about the hardest thing anyone can admit to in our culture! There are laws now that are called mental health parity laws that put mental health treatments on par (for insurance purposes) with physical medical issues. That's important! We really should see these struggles as something akin to medical problems. After all, depression IS a MEDICAL problem and what's more, it physically hurts! it is as painful physically as many other medical issues. It affects our families, our jobs, our physical health as much as (or in some cases more than) many physical ailments. It is not a weakness to admit that you have depression, any more than it is a weakness to admit that you have rheumatoid arthritis! Yet many of us are defensive about this like no other issue in life!

The problem with all that is that people who are depressed need to get treatment! If you are depressed your treatment is as important as treatment for a bacterial infection! It is like drowning and not calling out to the folks on the beach because you are embarrassed that you can't swim! And those of us on the beach or the dock are sipping our iced tea and looking passed the flailing masses, watching them drown while secretly hoping they don't look directly at us or ask for our help! They might see similar symptoms in us! (God forbid!)

The result of all this is that our culture judges people who have depression rather than seeing this for the huge medical problem that it is! All my life I have struggled with obesity and felt more times than not that I was flailing in the water, barely able to keep my chin above the water's edge. I was so embarrassed that someone might find out that I can't swim, I never wanted to ask for help! No matter what I did obesity was always there. Even gastric bypass surgery could not permanently rid me of this terrible disease! Nothing I did was ever enough! Certainly nothing was a cure.

In my experience obesity and depression are cousins of a sort. Someone said once that depression was anger turned inward. I see now why I wanted to eat more and not less when being told I was getting fat. In effect, the person telling me I was eating too much was pointing out a flaw in me. To that point as a child I never really thought of myself as being particularly flawed. I never thought I was perfect either. Those concepts had simply never entered my mind. But when I was first told that I was gaining weight and that I should eat less, I became aware that I was flawed. That made me embarrassed because prior to that point in my life I had never thought about food as any anything but sustenance. I never thought of it as something I had to pay attention to. I never really thought of it at all. I was hungry so I ate. My relationship with food was simple until then.

But embarrassment turned to anger at myself for not being perfect and I drove that anger inward forming a type of low grade depression and a life long disappointment in myself. And if I had obesity it seemed like the whole world new I wasn't perfect! It was like I thought I should have known better or something. It was clearly "my fault" that I was getting fat and I had no idea as a kid that hormones, genetics, disease, or inactivity played any role in this process at all. And there were people in my life with less than pure motives who were secretly glad for my stumble into obesity. Another problem in our culture. When we see someone else falter, sometimes we secretly rejoice because it is an unspoken, automatic step up the social rung for us. They would say things like, "It's really too bad you are overweight. You could be so pretty if you were skinny!" First, without even knowing it, those people publicly solidified my identity with obesity with those kinds of repeated and very public statements. It still amazes me that people who speak with authority, even when they don't know what they are saying, get the kind of credibility that they do. And it equally amazes me that we care so much about the opinions of people who do not have our best interests at heart. I knew those people weren't saying those things to positively motivate me. I knew that they were mean spirited people from all their other mean behaviors. Yet I took their nasty remarks to heart and continued to beat myself up over them for decades to come. I turned my anger inward and I ate.

The endorphins released by the experience of overeating did their job and temporarily made me feel comforted. I could have easily been cutting myself and gotten the same amount of physical comfort, but eating is so much more socially acceptable and nearly undetectable as a form of self abuse. Plus I don't like blood. But it isn't undetectable, is it? The results are there for all to see. Obesity is a public disease that is impossible to hide. And so we see the prejudice and harsh judgments that keep those with obesity from getting good jobs, raises, dates, and a whole host of other social advantages. And it is not just thin folks who judge us! We judge one another too! No group is innocent in this social crime.

So why is obesity like a half hearted suicide attempt? Because you don't really want to die. An unsuccessful suicide is not a coincidence, it is a cry for help. It's all about the methods people choose. People who are desperately in need of affirmation, acceptance, and positive experiences in life cry out in one way or another for help. We all want to know that it is ok that we aren't perfect. Self destructive behaviors are similar, no matter what form they take. Eating an entire bag of potato chips and dip is the same cry for help that cutting yourself or attempting suicide is. It just takes a more socially acceptable form. And far more people engage in food abuse than in other forms of self mutilation.

Depression can manifest itself in different ways in different people's lives. I'm not saying that just because you have obesity that you are automatically depressed. But I am saying that obesity is hard to live with in our society and it can cause depression. And obesity can be caused by depression too.

My point is that over eating is self harm. We are no better than the desperate kid who cries for help by cutting herself. Until we can see how self destructive our obesity inducing behaviors and ineffective coping strategies are, we will never get to their root causes. Do what is right by your body and it will respond in kind. If you continue to use food to cope with fear and pain, you will never resolve your emotional issues. It is at best a stop gap strategy and simply replaces short term emotional pain with long term physical pain. Ultimately you lose either way.

Like everything else we have talked about in this book, this is as individual as your diet and exercise needs. Awareness is critical. Search your self, be honest with yourself and be sure that you are not depressed, and then rest easy in that knowledge. But if you are depressed, please please get medical attention. It is ok that you are not perfect. You are in very good company.

Write Your Story

Create a journal entry this week about the most painful events of your life. Write them out in detail. I know this is difficult and I am sorry for that.

Now imagine yourself in those situations today, as an independent, secure, healthy adult. Write another account of the same event but this time instead of being caught unaware, you are ready for what's coming.

How would you react to the same event knowing what you know now? Write it with these advantages in your corner.

If you were a child, you are now an adult and you can respond to the event in a way that defends your younger self. Write the story the way you would experience it as an adult who knows exactly what's coming.

Write the kind of resolution you would have liked to have happened.

Create a scene where you win, you stop the pain before it happens, and you are whole and unhurt as if it never happened at all. Walk out of the scene knowing you were clever enough to stop the bad thing before it could cause you pain. How do you feel?

Now if you still need to resolve things with the people involved in those painful events, find a positive way to deal with those emotions. For example, you could write them a letter telling them how you feel and how you suffered at their hands. Don't mail the letter! The therapeutic value is in the writing! Be aware that if you decide to mail the letter you will probably get an unpleasant reaction. Maybe a very unpleasant reaction. There is a very real risk that you could be hurt further.

The idea is to process the pain, not make it worse! And this is not about revenge. This is about healing. If you do this with an eye to healing and freeing you from pain, revenge can have no part in it. You would get far more therapeutic value from ceremonially saying a few words and then burning the letter. As you watch the flames swallow the letter imagine the event melting away and let go as the smoke rises and then dissolves into the air.

CHANGES

One of the biggest deterrents to health for people who suffer with obesity is change. One change in your life can derail all your good life choices. The only thing to do is to fight fire with fire. Life is about change, and unfortunately most of us do not handle change with much success. It takes our well planned life and shakes it up, exposing us to all kinds of Temptation and making things that were finally easy, difficult again.

Two of the hardest hit areas in this war are Consistency and Schedule. Suddenly you must move across the country, or even across town and your whole exercise schedule, menu planning and journaling activities go up in flames. A death in the family or among your friends has the same kind of effect. Divorce or a job change are similarly powerful derailing forces. The change might be a change in someone in your family. Maybe your teenager is getting into trouble causing the whole family to unravel.

The idea here is to understand that these things are coming. Maybe you won't be able to see all of them coming, but certainly some of them. There is nothing we can do about change. But we can learn to manage it in ways that are healthier. How is that possible when we have no idea what changes are coming? Well rather than wait for it to hit and just react to it blindly, take some time to make plans. Plan for these changes so that when they happen you have something you can go to that will help you minimize the damage to your health.

I am not talking about some kind of internal contingency plan that is half baked. Change is coming. It will challenge your health. I promise you that. Not planning in advance for change is one of my biggest regrets in life.

When I was running and at the peak of health it never dawned on me that I could lose my ability to run. It was my "lifetime sport" and I was very happy doing it daily. Then I got sick and RA made it more and more painful to jog until I had lost all the cartilage in both knees and could no longer run at all. Just walking was (and is) painful. As I experienced this change in my practices, combined with medications like steroids, the weight piled on. I had no plan for what to do if I could not run. I was in so much pain I ended up in bed a lot. My docs were no help. And I loved running so much that the emotional component of losing that activity was (to me) similar to losing a good friend. The whole while I was begging my psychologist for help, I was trying really hard to figure out how to get back to my healthy practices. But that door had closed for me. I was grieving and I had no idea what to do because I had not made a contingency plan. I had not planned for change.

I have seen change derail myself and many others over the years. Don't let it derail you. Make a plan today. Look at your successful practices. What if you were no longer able to take part in them? What would you do instead? I should have begun to walk or swim, or anything to keep my fitness up. But I was so caught off guard I couldn't think about that. That's where a good plan comes in! If you have a plan you can go to when changes occur, you are more likely to weather the storm and get back to healthier practices more quickly than if you had no plan. During a crisis or a life change have a plan ready that you can go to without having to think about it. Create contingency plans for all your successful behaviors. And if you are married, plan for what you would do if your partner dies. Write these plans out. Keep them handy. This is a way you can show yourself love and compassion in those times when you will need it the most. Change will come. You may as well be ready for it.

Just to give you an example, my list of healthy practices includes daily movement. I have seasonal plans and backups for my exercise practices. Here in Washington it gets slick outside in the mornings during the winter months. This makes walking more difficult for me, given the hills here. Falling would really derail me. So, in the winter months I swim at a local gym which charges me $37 a month. I was able to look at my budget and stop buying coffee at cafes and pay for the gym membership that way. If I buy 10 lattes at cafes in a month, I am spending about $50. In fact, I could just buy a small plain coffee each time and save $30 toward the membership! If I had to stop swimming for some reason my plan is to drive to the nearest mall and walk indoors.

Write Your Story

What is your seasonal plan for exercise?

What are your plans when and if your seasonal exercise plans fail?

Now think bigger. Think about what you would do if you no

longer had your income, or a life partner? What if you were suddenly fired or laid off from a job you loved? How would you get through it? Would it derail your healthy practices?

Make a plan for the things in your life that are working. Then make a contingency to be able to continue to move forward in your quest for vitality if the worst should happen. Having a plan won't take away the pain of change. But it can make recovery a bit easier.

NOTHING MORE THAN FEELINGS

One of the first big insights my husband shared with me after we got married was that emotions brought on by hormones did not have to have associated meaning. This is profound. It meant that some emotions could simply be emotions, meaningless and harmless. It means that we don't have to assign meaning to emotion if we choose not to. Some emotions are driven by events in our lives, but many are simple physical reactions. If we could separate these kinds of physically triggered emotions from the nearly random meanings we attach to them, we might be able to conquer at least some emotional eating triggers. Consider the differences between emotion driven by events and emotion driven by hormones and other physical changes. (This applies equally to men and women, by the way.) We all have highly charged emotionally taxing events. These are things we must learn to manage as much as our physically driven emotions. I just had one yesterday, which prompted me to write this chapter. I dislike those days so much because I have lived my whole life acting on knee jerk reactions during those times. But yesterday was different. Yesterday I got some bad news, and you know what that's like. Something unexpected comes up and it isn't good. We've all been there many times. My bad news was that my doctor added another co-morbidity to my already long laundry list of disorders and diseases that I must fight and or manage. That was frustrating, but since there is no cure I knew it was worthless to dwell on it. So I was coping pretty well to that point.

Then I got hit with a double whammy. Wouldn't you know!? I got home from the doctor's office to an email about my PhD work. I was told I needed to do a pilot study before my primary study which would be set back at least another month, probably a lot more. (Turns out the change was really good for my research and I am glad for it!)

The long and short of it is that because of the double whammy I had just received I found myself in one of those highly charged emotionally difficult moments.

I was angry, I was frustrated, I even cried. All perfectly suitable reactions to the news of the day. Then I found myself moving toward my normal knee jerk reaction to highly frustrating situations and for the first time in my life I stopped. I didn't want the "comfort" of KFC chicken. It wasn't a will power thing at all. No more forcing myself to avoid my old coping mechanisms. I sincerely did not WANT to get KFC. The former comfort that KFC had provided me all those years seemed hollow and meaningless. I almost couldn't believe it myself! Those strong cravings, the emotional tug of the KFC family picnic were just gone.

I sat in silence for a few minutes enjoying the view from my newly acquired perspective. But what now? What do I do? What should I do to make myself feel better?

I saw this as an amazing opportunity to build a new coping skill. I was determined to make it something good for me, both physically and emotionally. I needed to let those emotions out, somehow process them. The tears were a good start. Since my husband was unavailable I picked up the phone and called my best-ie, and she was great! She was empathetic, supportive, and reminded me of the positive things about the situation, but not in a super sweet preachy way.

I'm very lucky to have people in my life that I can talk to at a moment's notice when I need support. It is worth building and committing to those relationships. Another contingency plan for when things go 'south' is to have a few people you can go to in a crisis and talk things through.

During the height of my emotional turmoil I did not reach for food. By the time I was actually hungry later that evening I had processed my emotions and I was clear headed enough to make good food choices. I think it is important to mention here that I was still kind of raw, emotionally. Because of that I chose a vegan lentil soup for dinner. It was perfect. Warm, soothing, healthy, and had all the right vitamins and nutrients to help my body cope and recover from an emotionally tough experience. Lentils are fat free, high in iron, B vitamins, fiber, and protein - namely tryptophan, which relaxes you! That's the substance in turkey that is responsible for the all-American Thanksgiving Nap! In addition, I added Turmeric which is used in many cultures as a pain killer. B vitamins have an amazing calming effect on emotions. I have used B vitamins in this way for years. I never stopped to think before this time how important it might be to my emotional recovery to eat something high in B vitamins when I am stressing. And It worked just as I had hoped!

Write Your Story

Make a plan for coping for the next stressful situation you

encounter. You don't have to know what will happen to plan for it. What will you do?

Choose something non-food related and practice doing it when you are not stressed. Keep this handy, like on a post it near your computer. That way when the stress hits you have your plan sitting right in front of you, reminding you to employ it.

Then the next time you are in a stressful situation stop and write down your plan for recovery. I know it is unnatural to do this, but that is the point. It might just bring a level of awareness that could stop harmful behaviors before they happen.

Notice your own knee jerk reactions. What are they? Take note of the trigger.

How commonly does this kind of thing happen to you?

How successful were you in employing your new strategy? Were you able to think before acting? If not, why?

What happened to derail you?

Send your stories to me, I would love to read them! carrieon@mac.com

WALK TOWARD THE LIGHT

When you dieted in the past you were always asked to walk away
from your old habits, your old patterns, old ways of doing things,
your old life. Unfortunately, the only "new life" that was being
offered was a purely physical one. We know that dieting is not just
a physical phenomenon. If it was simply physical, the disease of
obesity would have been cured decades ago. The trouble with that
physical philosophy is that we don't eat for simply physical reasons.
We know that. And so we are left to fend for ourselves running
headlong away from the old life into utter darkness. Once in the
darkness we are suddenly alone... cold... directionless. It is there
that we begin to doubt.

This is uncharted territory, completely unfamiliar to us. We
scramble about at first, trying to latch on to anything familiar,
anything that can help us on our way. We know we don't want to go
back to the old life, we swear to anyone and everyone we know that
we will never go back to the old fat self we have been. But the
darkness is way too scary and we are far too alone and worst of all
we have no idea how to live there. We no longer know who we are.
And no amount of cheerleading, rebuking, or platitudes can save us
from this unfamiliar and frightening darkness.

One of the most frequent "answers" to this problem in the diet
community is to exchange one compulsion for another. So, if you
are a compulsive overeater, then you need to exchange that
compulsion for a "better" one. The idea is that since they don't
know how to "cure" compulsive behaviors, they believe that you
must become a compulsive over-exerciser to keep yourself from
being a compulsive overeater. My bariatric surgeon even said to me
just after surgery, "Carrie, I know you will succeed because you are
compulsive."

The problem with that approach is that at the end of the day you are still compulsive.

Rather than working through the compulsivity, you simply ignore the problem altogether. Rather than finding out why you are compulsively eating, just shift your bad behavior pattern onto something better. For the vast majority of us, that's still not a solution. It is only a tiny minority of people who have been able to create for themselves almost by accident, a new identity based completely on a newly created dysfunctional behavior pattern. Most of them end up working (compulsively) in the weight loss, diet or fitness industry. Many become diet or fitness gurus whose only qualification is that they are "living proof" that what they did works. Never mind the fact that many are still secretly white knuckling it every day. Never mind the ones who feel deep down like impostors in their own lives who use cigarettes or other addictions to shove down the dysfunctional patterns that creep up daily. Never mind those who feel like if they ever stopped, even for a second, they would fall prey to their old lives and all that they have worked for would be gone.

But what about those of us who don't want to live life as a compulsive "anything"? What about those of us who want to focus on other aspects of our lives, like family and or career? What about balance? Wholeness? Being able to take a deep breath without fear of losing everything.

I propose a radical solution.

Walk into the light. Face it with all it's blinding brightness, and take one step after another until you have arrived at a new life. This new life is a place where you can see clearly who you are, how you got there, and how to live comfortably within it.

Breathe. Take a long, deep, satisfying breath. It will be a process, and there are no simple steps and no short cuts. But when you get there it will be worth it and best of all it will last for a lifetime.

The first thing we are going to do is to really get to know who we are. It's not just an inventory of what we eat. It's not a diary of revealing thoughts and anecdotes. It is so much better and more true than any of those could hope to be. We are going to research ourselves. Using some of the amazing free online tools that are currently available, we are going to find out where we are now, what we should eat, and what kind of exercise is best for our bodies! Amazing? Yup. When you put a personalized program together for yourself, you can see the evidence of your success. Add the psychological processes that lead to lasting change (which are detailed in this book) and you will succeed in the long term.

YOU GETTING TO KNOW... YOU

There is no one out there who knows you better than... you. And every single person on the planet is different from every other person. We all know that. So why on earth should we all fall in line with the latest, greatest diet plan?

It makes no sense that we would do anything but what is precisely right for us.

Individually.

But no one is going to create a plan, nor could they, that works perfectly for just you. Ok, until now. Now, using currently available technology, it is possible to study yourself without being a scientist or even a super brilliant science geek. These tools can be used to know more about where you are, from a fitness and health standpoint, right now. And they can be used to track how you feel when you eat a certain diet and give you precise information about what it is that you are eating that's stealing your energy. It can easily track and give you great feedback on how well you are progressing on a certain diet and or exercise program. Are you building muscle? How would you know? With current technology, it is possible to know.

I'm not talking about spending money here. All the tools I recommend can be used for free.

I know a lot of folks doing really well on a vegan diet. I know an equal number who do well on a high protein low carb diet, and some who love their paleo diet. I know that my friend Rosie can't eat the same diet I eat because the high number of greens would cause her intestines a lot of trouble. Some people have chosen a bariatric surgery diet, on account of having had the surgery. And for some of them it works wonders! I went for 5 years without eating one piece of fruit! Some people are like me and go between spending 9 months on a vegan diet and then a month or two on a low carb diet, and back to vegan... This about drove my kids a little crazy. Who can blame them? And I have to thank them (despite their endless teasing about this) for their support of me during those times. Not having the facts that are personalized for you can really be a head trip for some of us. I hate to admit how much I was tossed by the seas of indecision and confusion. But I am genuine and honest, never air brushed or phony. What you get isn't glamorous, but it is real.

I have no vested interest in which tool you use. I am not paid to recommend any given tool. If that ever happens, it would be because I truly believe in the tool and I would inform you of that decision up front. Transparency and accountability are important.

This is not just another diet program that you can imitate and experiment with, doing further damage to your metabolism. This is your program. Designed for you specifically. Not for you and your family. For you. Not for you and your sister or your best-ie, just for you. If you want to be told what and where to eat, and how to move, there are a lot of books that will spoon feed you that. But you know as well as I do that 98% of all diets fail. Why? Because they are not designed precisely and individually for you. They work precisely for the guru who designed the diet. But for 98% of the rest of us, they don't do the job!

And even if they do the job for a time and you lose weight, you are 98% likely to put it all back on and then some within a year! What a deal! At least you got to eat as much bacon as you wanted. <wry grin>

Work through the exercises in this book. Keep track of things using the program at the end of the book until you see results and patterns that help you to know what path works best for you.

LESSONS FROM WEIGHT LOSS SURGERY

If you read the first chapters you know that the inspiration for this book came from my PhD work with people who had weight loss surgery. The lessons I got from that experience are easily applied to weight loss in general. You don't have to have surgery to use the ideas that were borne out of that work. In fact, life is far easier if you haven't had surgery. I have mentioned that I had weight loss surgery in 2004. For the first five years it was amazingly successful. I lost 100 pounds and kept it off for those first five years. I was and still am grateful for the experience. Even though I ended up re-gaining my weight it fueled in me a desperate need to figure out what was happening. That led to my dissertation and this book. I am also grateful for the health and fitness levels that I enjoyed for those five years. It gave me a glimpse into the kind of authentic healthy life that I could live- IF I could maintain it.

That was of course, the problem. I couldn't maintain it. I did well as long as I could run 40-50 miles a week. Literally. That is 5 miles a day and ten miles each day on most weekends. But when I got sick and was diagnosed with RA, that changed overnight. I could no longer run... at all. I lost all the cartilage in both my knees in just two years and the process of that loss was very painful. My knee bones now rub together in a sort of super painful grinding action. Bone on Bone, they call it. It is as terrible as it sounds. I was told in 2010 after knee surgery that I needed knee replacement surgery, but that no surgeon would do it for at least another 20-25 years! Here's why many surgeons won't give artificial knees to young people, if you are curious. So, I was given some pain killers and told to do my best until then. Wow. That's not a very encouraging prognosis for the next 20-25 years.

So, I white-knuckled it for 4 years as I gained every single pound back, plus another 30 pounds! Talk about a recipe for depression! Seeing my fitness and health drain from my body week after week was devastating. I watched my pant size increase as I desperately scrambled to grab the last root, rock or vine on the edge of the cliff as I was dangling in mid air about to fall off.

Eventually I just fell. It was inevitable. No one can hold on forever. It is impossible. And it was as emotionally devastating as if I had fallen off a literal cliff. I was broken. Again. I thought that I had found the cure for obesity. I had lost the weight. I had kept it off for five glorious years. I was willing to do just about anything to keep the weight off. I had even said to my surgeon that I would have the surgery every five years if it meant keeping my health and size 4-6.

I did try that too! I went to the surgeon and asked about a "revision surgery". The problem was clear after an upper GI test showed that I had not stretched out my stomach or any part of the changed intestines so there was nothing to revise! I was still eating the same amount that I had for 5 years. I was still eating the same food I had for five years. But now I couldn't run 40-60 miles a week and that made all the difference.

I did try a variety of different RA friendly exercises. But those are hard to come by. Swimming was ok, but did not burn enough calories in the same time period that running did. So, I was spending literally half my day in the pool to maintain my calorie burn. That was not something I could do long term. I had a life, a family, a job, and all that comes with that. Walking is tough when your knees are rubbing bone on bone. Yoga was impossible since I couldn't get up and down off the floor several times in a workout. Anything that involved aerobics was simply too painful. Eventually I gave up.

It seemed to me that all I was left with was the side effects from the surgery, and no main effects. And the side effects are simply life altering. Don't get me wrong, I am grateful for these side effects in a way. They all lead to me eating better. But they are still difficult to deal with on a daily basis.

I have an intolerance for sugar that is quite severe. They call it dumping syndrome. It is a blessing in disguise for me, as it keeps me from eating large amounts of processed sugar. I can eat literally 6 grams of sugar (in a food that doesn't have substantial amounts of fiber or protein) without reacting to it. That's not much. I have a much lower tolerance for high fructose corn syrup (HFCS). That's right, it is NOT the same as sugar. If I eat ANY amount of it I "dump". It is very unpleasant and can lead to serious consequences if not dealt with immediately. It is in fact, Reactive Hypoglycemia. If I don't correct the imbalance in my blood sugar it will crash dangerously. I could potentially go into a diabetic coma. What happens is that when you eat sugar (or too much fat) it exits the stomach too early (not enough processing has gone on) and it hits a part of the intestine that absorbs it too fast and it goes into the blood stream more rapidly than it would in a person with a normal anatomy. The blood sugar spikes for a short time and immediately drops to levels that can be dangerously low. In the mean time you are dizzy, sweating, nauseated, blacking out, heart palpitations, and weakness. Not fun. If you eat a high protein snack that contains just a small amount of carbohydrates you can balance your blood sugar. But it takes time, and it is very unpleasant.

The problem isn't that people who have had weight loss surgery cheat and eat high sugar foods (it can be a problem but that is another whole story). The problem for well meaning, dedicated patients is that pre-processed foods contain so many ingredients that we don't yet understand, and that might be disguised by unfamiliar names, that we aren't always sure what we are eating. If you eat something that you assume has no sugar like spaghetti sauce, you may still dump because a lot of pre-prepared spaghetti sauces have not only sugar but High Fructose Corn Syrup or both! Who would have thought?

Needless to say, it forces you to become a well-educated, label reading consumer. That's a good thing.

There are some important principles about diet and exercise that I learned from my bariatric surgery experience. These are some of the rules they teach you about how to live after surgery. They are rules that could help anyone do better with food and exercise.

Eat Slowly.

With each bite, chew completely until your food is applesauce consistency. After each bite clear the mouth completely before taking another bite. To help you remember to do this, put your fork or spoon down between bites. The whole applesauce analogy sounds gross, but it is important to digestion. Many of us eat so fast that we barely take any time to chew. It has a negative effect on digestion when we basically cut out the first step in digestion which is processing food in your mouth. Thoroughly mixing our food with saliva is very important as it begins the breakdown of the food and the digestion process. When we do this, we are allowing our bodies to absorb much more of the nutrients in our food.

Do Not Drink While you are Eating.

If you drink while eating you flush the food through faster and you will feel hungry sooner. There is a second part of this rule. Do not drink for at least 20 minutes after eating. This is important for the same reason. And this gives your body more time to absorb the nutrients in your food before flushing it through the system.

Eat for Only 20-30 Minutes- But Eat for a minimum of 20 Minutes

Limiting the amount of time that you eat, coupled with eating more slowly is a recipe for weight loss, and lower calorie intake. But forcing yourself to take at least 20 minutes to eat one cup of food (the typical serving for someone after gastric bypass- if you haven't had surgery you may want to try 2 cups) is an amazing feat. It takes some practice with small bites, chewing very thoroughly, clearing your mouth completely between bites. This has an added effect that is important. It gives your stomach enough time to tell your brain that you are full BEFORE you have over eaten! Think of it! No more after meal misery, guilt, or remorse. Just a satisfied full sensation to take away from the table. And in case you feel emotionally weird about eating so little, just remind yourself that you will be eating again in 3 to 4 hours! You will be fine!

Eat Three Meals a Day

Eating three meals a day is important because so many people who have obesity are accustomed to skipping breakfast. Skipping breakfast sounds on the surface like a way to cut down on calories, but in fact what happens is that when lunch rolls around you ingest far more calories than if you had eaten breakfast and lunch. In addition, after weight loss surgery, you must eat within 45 minutes of waking in order to maintain a healthy blood sugar and insulin level. So three meals a day is important. Small high quality snacks may also be important.

Eat Every 3-4 Hours During the Day

Again, this is a blood sugar issue. It is a way to keep insulin levels even and consistent. But it is not a license to eat 5 meals a day. What it means is that you need just 50 or 100 calories in between meals if your meals are more than 4 hours apart. High quality small snacks are the key.

Be Mindful While You Eat

This one is self evident. Think about your choices and how they are (or are not) going to nourish your body. Don't focus on satisfaction, or taste as much as nutrient content. The satisfaction and taste will take care of itself.

If You Are Not Dripping Sweat- You Are Not Exercising

This is a BIG ONE! It sort of stunned me at first. I thought that going for a walk was exercise until I heard this. Well it is not exercise unless it causes you to literally drip sweat. And it might! But for many people a simple stroll isn't going to cause the dripping sweat necessary to be considered rigorous enough to be real exercise. This also will help you to regulate the amount of time you exercise. If you know that a minimum of 30 minutes of exercise a day is good for you, you must workout until you begin to drip sweat. Then you can begin to count your 30 minutes. And remember, that is a minimum. If you want to lose weight, or maintain weight loss your requirements may be much more than that. I found a minimum of one hour a day was necessary to keep my weight off. That was my minimum. Not my ideal. Just the bare minimum. Having the disease of obesity means that your minimums are going to be higher than what someone who doesn't have this disease needs to do. You have a disease. Start to manage it like a disease.

My sweet husband is fond of saying that exercise is wasted energy (our oldest son Noah came up with the idea). He means that in the most positive, literal way possible. If you are walking and you get to your destination, you have not wasted energy. You have simply used the minimum required energy to get to where you are going. That's not exercise. If however, if you jog to your destination, you are using more energy than would be required to simply arrive at the destination. Therefore, you are wasting energy. That is exercise. When he went to purchase his bicycle a year or two ago he shocked the salesperson by asking for a bike that would be more difficult to pedal. The bike salesperson was taken aback. He'd never heard that before. Everyone else in his experience had always asked for bikes that made it easier to get from point A to point B. But Steve wanted it to be as difficult as possible, so that he could be sure he was expending as much energy to ride the bike as possible. After all, that was why he was getting a bike- for exercise!

Drink A Lot of Water Every Day

Fat exits the body primarily in two ways: through your sweat or through urine or both. How can you expect to lose fat if you have not created a way for it to exit the body? We must encourage the body to let go of fat, and in this simple action we are giving it free passage out. So drink lots of water, and do REAL EXERCISE every day.

These life lessons are applicable to anyone whether you have had surgery or not. They will help lower caloric intake, absorption of nutrients, and elimination of stored fat from the body. What could be better?! These rules help contribute to the long term success of weight loss surgery. But they could help you to keep your weight off forever too.

Having said all that, weight loss surgery clinics although well-meaning, still do not adequately address the psychological issues surrounding weight loss maintenance. The best I have seen are clinics that provide therapist guided support groups. These support groups can be very good, or they can be like a few that I attended early on. The bad ones meet at restaurants, and eat while they are supporting one another. So, once a month (or even once a week in some cases!) they eat processed, high salt, high fat, and high sugar laden food that is probably the least ideal to support their needs as a person with the disease of obesity. These are foods that should almost never be eaten by someone with this disease!

However, all the support groups I have been to have one very very big problem in common. When weight losers get together for support most often what they are struggling with comes up in discussion. It is natural to confess how you've cheated throughout the last week or month because that is what you want support in avoiding next week. While it may be cathartic for the person who is confessing their "food transgressions" it is for the non-cheaters a type of education in how to get around the rules! It gave me ideas for "cheating" I would never have had on my own!

The problem with all of this is that the research about weight loss maintenance clearly states that when people attend support groups they are far more likely to maintain their weight loss. What?! Now I know I need support on a regular basis, but the support groups I went to did not fulfill that need for me. It's like a whole group of diabetics getting together every week to talk about how they can manipulate their insulin shots in order to eat more chocolate cake.

I think the solution is a saner version of support. Make some very basic ground rules (don't over do it) about what kinds of things are shared. Maybe the details of the cheat don't have to be disclosed. Saying anything that might make someone else stumble, intentionally or otherwise, is not supportive. Be mindful that you are there for yourself, but also for the others in the group. Break the cultural norm of meeting around food. Even if you meet at meal time, don't feature food at or after your meetings. If you take care of yourself, eat a small snack or early dinner before the meeting, it will probably not go more than 4 hours giving you the window you need not to eat during that time. Provide water or unsweetened, caffeine free herbal tea. We all need to drink more water. Reinforce the things you know work to help you and the others in your group manage this disease.

But make no mistake, this is a small part of the equation. This is just the physical stuff. Without the psychological processing, this is as temporary and meaningless as every other diet you've ever been on. And better you should learn the lessons of weight loss surgery without having the surgery!!

Write Your Story

Have you ever considered weight loss surgery? (or wondered what life would be like for you after weight loss?)

Of the lessons from weight loss surgery, what are you presently doing that works for you?

What have you tried of these suggestions that has not worked?

Do you think these techniques are valuable?

What, if any, of these techniques will you incorporate into your life?

How will you know if they work for you or not?

Decide up front what success looks like with regard to each of these techniques. If you don't know what success looks like, how will you know when you get there?

Monitor your changes after incorporating one technique at a time (no more than one change per week) into your life. If you incorporate more than one technique per week you will not know which one worked.

What are the results?

THAT 'NASTY' PLATEAU

You may think you know what I am about to tell you about weight loss plateaus, but you would probably be wrong. The current concept, in case you are unfamiliar, is that when we lose weight our body becomes too used to our current routine and we stall out at certain points, stop losing weight and "plateau" for a time before losing weight again. Many people are completely frustrated by this, and I was too. That is until I decided that we are looking at this process all wrong. Please understand, I know that the phenomenon happens. I have been through it many times. But the idea that your body is "stalled out" or your weight loss process has stopped is the wrong way to see it. Plateaus are a vital part of the weight loss process and should be seen as such.

When we lose weight we do get to those places where the scale seems to stand still for days, weeks, even months. But it isn't stalling out at all. It is simply your body adjusting to the recent radical changes, and preparing itself for more change. Think about what you have done when you begin to lose weight. You change the way you eat, your body is moving more, the weight loss itself means that the body has lost something it was used to. It takes some assimilation for your body to make these changes last. This isn't a negative thing at all, it is all about incorporating these radical changes into your body's new "normal".

Without plateaus these changes might be more difficult for us to sustain. If we simply lost weight without plateaus our bodies and our minds would have a lot more to adjust after arriving at our goal weight. This way, the body takes it a step at a time, gradually incorporating the changes so that we can get accustomed to our bodies as they become healthier, stronger, and more fit.

On a molecular level, your body is changing all the time. New cells are being produced, old ones sloughing off. They say that over a period of seven to ten years a lot of the cells in our bodies renew themselves. There are some types of cells that we are born with like heart muscle cells, cells in the inner portion of the crystalline lens of our eyes, and in the brain the cerebral cortex neurons. But the experts tell us that most of our other cells change and renew over time. We get a new skeleton approximately every ten years. So what are we doing to support that new skeleton over the next ten years?

Will you develop osteoporosis in the next ten years or will you support the renewal of your bones with weight bearing exercise and sufficient daily calcium and vitamin D intake?

What does that mean for weight loss? It is important to know that with all those cellular changes, combined with changing our diets and exercise routines, we are asking a lot of our bodies. It only makes sense that we should be patient with those changes and the processes that lead to a healthier body, including plateaus. I'm not a biologist, but I imagine the body changing so radically during dietary changes that it might just need some time to slow the process down in order to assimilate all those changes and to continue to renew itself too.

Part of the reason that I bring this up is that in our culture (and many others) we want change to happen quickly. We have all seen the ads and books, "30 Days to a Thin Beautiful You!" "60 days to OMG!" Instant gratification is our way of life. We microwave our food, impatient that it might take two whole minutes to heat up dinner. Part of becoming an authentically healthy person is to recognize the different processes our bodies are going through and to sync up psychologically and emotionally with those processes, rather than always pushing for more weight loss faster. Take time to listen to your body. If your body needs some time to plateau, support that, enjoy it, take it as a positive sign that your body is assimilating the changes you are making to it and when you are ready in both body and mind to make more changes you will begin to lose weight again (assuming you still need to lose weight).

But push and rush through the process ignoring your body and you are sure to regain all the weight you have lost and probably more.

There is now no guilt for being in a plateau. It isn't a problem at all, certainly nothing you are or have been doing wrong. It is simply a part of the process of renewal. It is a gift from your body to remind you to take the time necessary to change on the inside to reflect those changes in your body. It is your body's way to allow you to sync up, be authentic and whole in body and in mind.

One last thought on plateaus. I don't see a plateau as a time when I have stopped losing weight. I see it as a time when I am learning to maintain the weight I have already lost. Weight loss maintenance is the difficult part. Keeping it off is the Holy Grail. Rather than being disappointed every time you get on the scale and it doesn't move downward, take joy in those opportunities you have been given to learn how to keep the weight off.

YOU: RE-IMAGINED

As teenagers we go through a time of extreme change from childhood to adulthood. This time in our lives is marked with both physical and emotional changes. These psychological and social changes are so well understood that inside the profession of psychology they have been well studied for decades by many now famous psychologists. The result of these severe and unsettling changes is that the teenager becomes a new person; their adult self. In our adolescence we allow these changes to happen in the most natural, instinctive ways. And for most people the process happens and the changes take place and they become independent, responsible adults who are equipped with a new more mature identity ready to take on the challenges of an adult life.

For many young adults obesity is part of that identity. However, obesity doesn't have to happen in the teen years for it to become part of your identity. For many who have the disease in adulthood, it does happen first in childhood. Even if you were told your whole life that you were fat when you weren't, you might still have taken that on as part of your identity. And it is kind of a "double whammy" if you will. Your initial identity is forming and in addition to becoming an adult there is the strong presence of a chronic, very public disease.

If you have the disease of obesity you can't hide it. Oh, you can try. We have all tried. Whole industries have been built on hiding obesity. Still, everyone who ever sees you, including strangers on the street, children, the educated and uneducated, the rich, the poor, everyone knows that you have it. It is inescapable. If you have the disease of obesity, it is by definition, part of your identity.

So why not deliberately use the same process that we use instinctively to change from children into adults to change our entire identity from fat and unhealthy to authentically healthy and whole? That was the question that sparked my dissertation study. Here's a bit of it:

"It is said that having weight loss surgery (WLS) is like being reborn into a newly created body (Bocchieri, Meana, & Fisher, 2007). Because of the dramatic changes made during and resulting from the surgery, the patient must learn to eat, drink, walk, sit, stand, and dress themselves all over again (J. Ogden & Clementi,

2010; Throsby, 2008). They must re-learn key social skills and assert themselves into new roles by relating in new ways to friends, parents, siblings, colleagues, mentors, bosses, mates or potential mates. Many celebrate the day of weight loss surgery as a new birth day (Bocchieri et al., 2007; Throsby, 2008). Just after surgery, the shaky patient, very much like a newborn baby, takes their first tentative sips of water into their tiny new stomach, and before they know it, their first steps into a brand new life with a brand new identity" (Hickman, 2012).

Weight loss surgery forces the patient to go through a true physical metamorphosis. That's why I chose that group of people to study weight loss maintenance. Like I have said, losing weight is easy. Keeping it off is the Holy Grail. Weight loss surgery has a much higher success rate for weight loss than any non-surgical weight loss method (Hall, 2010; Herpertz et al., 2003; Kushner & Noble, 2006; Netherton, 2008; Van Etten & Grimaldi, 2011). In fact, non-surgical weight loss has about a 2-5% success rate, while surgical weight loss success rates were 90% before 1995, by 2012 success rates are about 60% and dropping like a rock as more and more people have the surgeries.

By success I mean life long weight loss. I mean never gaining it back. Others may have another definition of success. I am sure that my bariatric surgeon thinks that my gastric bypass was successful. A surgeon's definition of a successful surgery is far from successful life long weight loss maintenance. After all, they are surgeons. By definition, if the surgery accomplished it's goal (re-routing your intestines) and you did not die during or immediately after surgery, it was a success.

But that is not my definition of a successful weight loss surgery. Not by a long shot. That is only the very first step in a long process that may or may not result in permanent weight loss and life long health. And it does not take into consideration the psychological, psychosocial, or the emotional side of this disease.

And generally speaking there is a considerable psychological component to weight loss. While that might ring true for some people, not every obese person has childhood abuse in their background. Some obese people had rather idyllic childhoods.

The process of unburdening yourself is an extremely important one, and many people need to do it. Psychologists and therapists are our greatest allies in our struggle to become whole.

However, that is still only part of the picture.

To their credit, many psychologists and therapists work to help us develop healthier habits. There is a lot of value in that for sure!

But if the disease of obesity could be resolved by building new habits, and we have all been told that it takes 30 days to build a new habit, why do so many people regain their weight after 2 or 3 or even 5 years? It's because weight loss maintenance isn't about new habits. It is about building a new identity.

You might be very satisfied with who you are, from a social standpoint. That's wonderful. We aren't talking about an introvert suddenly becoming the life of every party. We are talking about incorporating something into the successful and functioning parts of your personality. We are talking about changing from having an image of laziness and incompetence to success, vibrancy and health. You stay you. This is just you with your shine on!

How do you build a new identity? Well it is about time to get to the heart of it.

ERIKSON

In 1963, Erik Erikson formulated a theory about how we transform from life as children to life as adults. He didn't stop after adolescence was vanquished. His theory continues on throughout the human lifespan. Erikson's theory explains exactly how we navigate through eight different stages in life to first develop our identity and then to live authentically throughout our lives within that identity. It is upon the bedrock of Erikson's theory that I have built my own theory. The individual tasks are slightly different, but the goal of an authentic, whole, satisfying, and healthy life could not be more closely aligned with Erikson's theory.

And it is important you know that Erikson's theory of psychosocial development has been tested, studied, and verified down to the last jot and tittle. That's important. This is an accurate description of how we develop over our lifespans.

Psychosocial development is just a fancy way to say that while you are maturing psychologically, your social interactions are maturing too. Psycho-social. The reason that is important for us is that developing a new healthy identity doesn't just involve us. It intimately involves all the people in our lives, both significant and insignificant.

Many diet and exercise gurus focus solely on the person who wants to lose weight. A few might even include the family and friends of that person, asking them to "encourage" or not to sabotage their friend as they lose weight. But that is as far as I have ever seen any guru go. And it just isn't enough.

When you were a teenager there was not a single relationship in your life that wasn't effected by your adolescent development. Suddenly you hated your mom, your friends came in and out of favor. Your father simply had no clue. Everyone in your life was faced with a decision. Either they allowed their relationship with you to change, or they dropped off the map. Friendships changed, your relationships with family members changed, some friends dropped off and new ones came into the picture. But no one was immune to those changes. The same is true for building your new, healthy, authentic identity. Those people who are not good for you, who continually sabotage you, who don't respect your choices, may end up falling off the map. Things like this have to happen for you to truly change. This is not just a psychological change. It is a social change too.

I'm reminded of the old psychology joke:

Q: How many psychologists does it take to change a light bulb?

A: One, but the light bulb must be willing to change.

You don't live in a vacuum, and the changes you make won't happen in a lab somewhere. They happen in real time, in your life. That life is filled with friends, parents, children, mates, co-workers, etc. And your relationships with them shape and reinforce your choices in life.

Your job is to work through each of these eight stages of development in order to build a new healthy, authentic, satisfying and self-consistent life. These stages will be presented in the next chapters. Journals, worksheets, and questionnaires will accompany these pages so that you are not simply an observer in this process, going through the motions, mimicking the guru (so to speak). If you work through them, process the information and apply it to your life and your commitment, you will see that just as you worked through adolescence, you will become the person you always wanted to be.

When I got sick and began to gain weight I went to a psychologist, someone I respect very very much, and pleaded with her to help me stop the onslaught of weight gain. I had gone through the extreme pain of gastric bypass and was determined to keep the 100 pounds I'd lost, at bay. She could do nothing to help me! She knew that if I worked on my "issues" I would be more mentally healthy, and that would help me in general. But that was all she could offer. Nothing specific to weight gain. Nothing specific to deal with the terrible prospect of losing my hard fought weight loss battle! The weight-gain-inducing medications, the lack of exercise and generalized frustration all caused me to regain the 100 pounds I'd lost, plus some! So, there I was with the side effects of gastric bypass, but none of the "main effects"!

What I mean to say is that if I ate too fast, or something too dry, the food would get stuck in the very tiny opening to my stomach and caused at least an hour of what felt like a heart attack! If I ate too much sugar or fat, I "dumped" for at least an hour. Dumping is basically profuse sweating, severe nausea, and then diarrhea that lasts at least an hour. Sugar can create a reactive hypoglycemic reaction that can be deadly. I passed out twice from low blood sugar in the first two years after surgery. I will admit, some of these side effects are actually good for me. I don't want to eat too much sugar or fat. It's great that my body doesn't tolerate them. I am actually grateful for that. But getting "stuck" is a difficult thing to be grateful for. And having these restrictions, along with a one cup stomach, that could help you stay thin was a price I readily paid. The problem was that having those restrictions without the benefit of the "main effect" of staying thin became a real bummer!

Unfortunately 40% of all people who have gastric bypass are just like me! And that number rises every year! They lose the weight, and regain it back (and usually more) within a couple years! If I was an isolated case, it would be tragic for me. But the problem is that I am far from an isolated case! The surgery is failing more and more people every year! The more people who have the surgery (this includes lap band surgeries too!) the higher the percentage of people we see regaining the weight. Why is it that so many more people seem to be in this category now than 20 or 30 years ago?

It's actually very interesting. Before 1991 the rules for gastric bypass were very strict. The surgery was reserved for patients who had extreme morbid obesity. These were people you heard about on the news who were 400+ pounds and had to be buried in piano cases. The surgery wasn't considered an alternative for people who were not in this extreme category, and very few people had the surgery. It was performed only as a last ditch effort to save the life of the person when all else had failed and death seemed imminent without it. For those few it was relatively successful. Follow up care was much more intense, and for some of these people it seemed to work.

Fast forward to 1991. There was a big conference of The American Society of Metabolic and Bariatric Surgery during which some key recommendations were made regarding who should qualify for bariatric surgery. One of the recommendations was to extend or open the qualifications to those who have a BMI of 30 to 40 as long as they also had co-morbidities. We have already talked about how common co-morbidities are with obesity. Still, most patients were at a BMI 40 or more because that was the new threshold without co-morbidities. And as a result of this new ruling in 1991, the flood gates had opened!

Let's examine what that means. First, a BMI of 30 translates to a woman who is 5'3" and 170 pounds. Or a man who is 5'11" and 215 pounds. This opened up the option for gastric bypass and other weight loss surgeries to people who had previously not qualified. A lot of people. And because of the recommendations made in the ASMBS conference, insurance was now paying for it! Is it any wonder that there was a huge influx of weight loss surgeries that began in 1991? Suddenly if you had high blood pressure and carried just over the recommended amount for a "healthy weight" and had good health insurance you were a candidate for weight loss surgery. Many many people who would previously have never considered it were standing in line waiting (some for a year or more) for their turn to be cut open and made magically thin! Me included!

The reality of it is that no matter how you lose weight, whether by surgery or by sheer willpower, you still need to deal with the psychological issues that are ever present, and that threaten to upend any and all progress you have made toward a healthier lifestyle. This is precisely why weight loss maintenance is the Holy Grail. No one out there has yet to tell you how to truly change your life forever! Until now.

The question boils down to, if even something as extreme as weight loss surgery isn't a cure, how can I hope to lose weight and keep it off? The answer is in understanding permanent health change. These eight stages are your gateway to changing not only your lifestyle, but your entire identity. And that, my friend is the key to success.

YOUR NARRATIVE

Everyone has a story. You have a story, and so do I. But contrary to what most people believe, your story is completely within your control. You decide what the story of your life will be. Each day, every hour you spend living it, every choice you make builds your narrative. And in the final assessment of your life, what will be left is your story. How you lived, who you were, what you did and said will be left as a record. This is the evidence of who you were and what and who you cared about. What will that evidence tell others about you when you can no longer speak for your self?

You may think that only people who write books tell stories. But you would be wrong. Your life tells the story of you. What is your Personal Lore? What knowledge and experience do you have to share with the world? What can the world learn from your life?

Every day that you live is a new page, a new adventure. Sometimes there are twists and turns, sometimes sorrow, sometimes overwhelming joy. Who you are is what the unfolding story reveals. Each time you overcome an obstacle, your story deepens. With each setback, your image clears just a bit more. You get to know who you are through these plot twists in your life, and so do those who share your life.

What are you known for? What is the image you project to the world? Who are you? It's a tough question that can't be answered with a simple sound-byte. That's part of what makes diseases so difficult to fight. They become such a big part of our identity that it is difficult for us to change and for others to 'allow' us to change.

You may have noticed that I try hard not to refer to people (or myself) as fat people, or obese people. I hope never to say, "I am obese" again. That's not because I have lost weight and I hope never to gain it back again. It's not about that. And I'm not in denial. Quite the contrary. I want to be accurate. If I say that I AM obese, I am telling you that it is an integral part of who I am. It then becomes further embedded in my mind that a part of my identity (who I am) is obesity. And since obesity is such a public affliction, saying that aloud reinforces the idea that I AM OBESE (and all that entails) in the minds of others. In turn, that reinforces in my own mind that obesity is part of my identity. That's how people get nicknames like Fat Albert. By the time you've gotten the nickname of "Tiny" because you are so large, it is completely cemented in your brain and the brains of your friends, and anyone you introduce yourself to, that obesity is a part of who you are.

That just should not be. And it can be turned around, if we make the choice to reject that notion and change our language. That's the first step in changing your story. And it is an important one.

But just like companies manage their brands, you must manage your narrative. Because your narrative is constantly evolving and changing with time and experience, it is vital that you make choices that will help build the narrative that you want to build. You are not a helpless victim in this life. No matter the hardships, you can direct your reactions.

"I grew up in a relatively poor household. Like a lot of people we didn't really know we were poor..." That's how my narrative begins. There's pretty much nothing you can do about the circumstances of your upbringing, and they are (for most people) not a credit to your intelligence or goodness either. They simply are. So drop it. Start your narrative now. I mean right now, inside your own head. Positive self talk is one of the most powerful things we can do to ensure our success. And the converse is true too. When your self talk revolves around not feeling good, mentally or physically, it ensures that your narrative will follow suit. It must. So think about the way you think about yourself, your situation, and your life. Is it positive? Hopeful? The old phrase "count your blessings" is a way to begin. I don't want you to lie to yourself or to act in denial of your basic situation. But everyone can think of something about their life to count as a blessing. What is in your heart will soon come out of your mouth too.

What do you talk about with strangers you meet on the bus or in the bank while you wait? What are the first few topics that usually come up? This will give you your first clues to your narrative and to what's important to you. No matter what the circumstances, the things that are important to you always seem to make their way into conversation. What do you talk about with your hair dresser? This may seem trivial but it is very telling. I usually talk about my family, my writing, my PhD work. For me, those represent the cream that rises to top of my mind in situations where I don't really know the person well, but we talk every month or two.

Think about your last conversation with your hair dresser or barber. Maybe you talk periodically with the guy who changes your oil. What did you talk about? Did you talk about the others in your life to the exclusion of anything about you? Or did you share something about yourself? A recent trip you took? The progress you are making on a goal you are working toward? Think about it because it is a reflection of who you are and what you care about. Do you take care of everyone but yourself? It will be reflected in the way you talk to others about your life. When someone asks you 'what's new?' what do you answer? Is your answer about your son or daughter going off to college and your husband's new job? What does it say about what's new with you? It is okay to talk about the others in your life, but this little observation will tell you something about what your true focus in life is. Are you focused on bettering yourself in some way? I find most people I ask the question 'what's new?' answer that there is nothing new at all in their lives. I know it isn't true, because their stories are not over.

Write Your Story

I want to challenge you to think about your answer to the question 'where are you in life right now?' Describe in detail you life as it is right now.

Make a timeline of the changes you would like to see in your life and when you would like to see them come to fruition.

How are you directing your own narrative?

What are you doing to make your life the best it can be? Make a list.

How are you planning to grow and change in the next 3 months, six months, a year?

We can all better ourselves. No one is perfect. How will you better the lives of those around you?

How will you insure your memory after your life is over?

What will people remember about you? What do you want them to remember about you?

Will people describe you as obese? Lazy? Incompetent? It is my experience (and research bears this out) that people who suffer with obesity are as much a cross section of society as people who do not have obesity. Ambition doesn't have a waist size. Nor does being lazy or incompetent. Obesity carries with it a heavy stigma. It's just reality. Fortunately, you can smash that stigma and shape your narrative so that what people know about you is that you are smart, funny, sexy, and vibrant or whatever you want to be. But it is your job to care enough about your narrative to shape it, and reshape it until it is what you want it to be. The steps in the following chapters will help you do just that.

STAGE ONE: TRUST

Trust must be absolute. There can be no flickers of doubt, no holding back. You either trust or you don't. Period. Newborns are given example after example of trustworthy behaviors from their parents, as with each distressing cry there is a response of food or change or comfort. This simple trust relationship is the cornerstone of stage one: Trust versus Mistrust. Today's diet landscape is nothing short of a minefield. Every month (or less) there's a new "diet breakthrough" that's going to end obesity! Low carb, grapefruit, hormone shots, raspberry keytones, you name it, it's out there! And it's all about money, not about curing the disease of obesity. (In case you missed any of these "earth shattering wonders" they don't work! Don't waste your money.)

"Eat like a Caveman! They weren't fat!" Each diet plan has their own logic, and that's what sucks people in. Never mind that Paleolithic man had to hunt sometimes for days, chase prey for miles, kill, skin, gut, clean, and cook all her own meat. All that and we don't really know if Paleolithic people were fat or not!

On many of these new diets people lose weight- at least at first. But there is always the flicker... doubt is always there in the back of your mind - even as you are dedicating yourself to yet another diet movement. Mistrust sneaks in through these flickers of doubt. Is this the "one diet for me"? From there daily evidence and observations fuel mistrust and it grows. Day by day it makes you restless, more and more unsure of what you are doing. Let me be clear, we will push our doubts aside in the name of results. But when the results falter, the questions re-emerge.

Questions emerge about the trustworthiness of the diet program. Important questions. Like, how is this diet going to affect my heart on a long term basis? How much do we know about the long term effects of this diet? Cave men only lived about 30 years or so. If I am supposed to stay on this for life, is it going to keep me healthy into my 90s? Is this really good for me? Couple all those mounting questions with the difficulty of the lifestyle, and your flicker becomes a flame! Once mistrust has a foothold, the new diet doesn't stand a chance. And frankly, more often than not that is a good thing.

This is your mind's way of telling you that you simply cannot take this diet as a part of your identity, because it has not proven itself trustworthy, and it is out of alignment with who you really are.

Doubt isn't a problem, and it is not an issue of you not committing yourself properly. It is a good thing that keeps you from going down paths that are not right for you. But it is one of the big reasons that 98% of all diets fail.

Think about that guy you dated in High School or college. At first you really liked him, he was a dream boat after all! But when you got to know him you started to have doubts about whether or not he was really right for you. His quirky immature behaviors seemed novel and cute at first, but long term they were destructive and non-productive. In High School he was the class clown, tons of fun. But in the real world that wears thin fast.

It's the same kind of thing. You dropped him because long term he wasn't someone you could commit to. He wasn't good for you. The two of you as a couple just weren't going to work. It may have been a painful time in your life, but it is easy in hindsight to see how breaking it off was the right thing to do.

All of these programs tell you now that you must take them as a lifestyle. That they are not a diet. That's right. But it isn't the whole story. And even if you find the perfect diet plan for you (which, by the way, may be the Paleo diet) they still do not tell you HOW to successfully psychologically integrate it into your life. All the menus and rules for eating and encouraging mantras and platitudes even bullying and threats can't help you to truly change long term.

You are still left with the mother load of the work! They give you all the parts of a car, and then tell you to put it together, learn to drive it, and operate it safely and maintain it on a day to day basis. But HOW? I don't know how to do that! I've never done it before, and I simply do not have the education, background or manual dexterity to assemble a car.

So there you are, standing in your driveway with all of the car parts strewn all around you, paralyzed. There's a fender to your left, some nuts and bolts in the grass, a couple tires have rolled to the end of the drive. You pick up the steering wheel, because that looks familiar and you hold it in front of you. It's brand new, shiny, and it fits nicely in your hands. For a few minutes it feels really good. As you stand there waiting for the car to materialize around you, you begin to wonder what those other parts are for. What do you do with them? They must be there for a reason, but you've never assembled a car. Now you are back to being paralyzed.

That's the level of guidance you get from diet plans. All the car parts are the psychological components of your life that are strewn about you unaddressed. You know that you need every one of them. And you need to figure out where every single part goes, but putting the whole thing together by yourself, making sure that it fits together as a complete whole seems impossible and quite frankly overwhelming.

And say just for the moment that you finally manage to put the entire car together, where do you fit in it? Do you fit in it? Or are you gripping the steering wheel so tight that your knuckles turn that familiar shade of white? You know what I mean. Even if you manage to assimilate yourself into the diet guru's world, it still may not be right for you. There still may be questions in the back of your mind about the whole thing. If there are questions, you will fail to navigate this first and very important stage of Trust versus Mistrust.

Unfortunately, that's as far as many of us get with diet gurus. It is not a failure on your part. I cannot emphasize that enough! Failing to navigate these stages is not a personal failure. It is simply a fact. This diet plan that you are attempting to trust isn't completely trustworthy. If it is a failure at all it is the failing of the program to be worthy of your trust. It is a failure because it is not worthy of becoming an authentic part of your life.

If you cannot eat gallons of cabbage soup every day for the rest of your life, it isn't a personal failure. That is ridiculous. The cabbage soup diet simply isn't worthy of becoming part of your identity.

How do you know before you take on a new diet that it isn't worthy of you? Try it on psychologically! Using the cabbage diet as an example: Are you "that person who devoted their life to cabbage"? Sounds extreme doesn't it?

The idea of devoting your life to cabbage might not bother you at first because of the short term results. After all, we are (many of us) so desperate to lose weight that we can and do ignore, at least for a time, the psychological associations with cabbage (or weight loss surgery, or Atkins, or whatever). But long term you know you are going to want to eat something other than cabbage. And that you will want a more balanced association with food. You may also want people to see you as more than the cabbage person with the gas problem (which of course is a trait of all cabbage people).

Please understand, I am not knocking cabbage, or the paleo diet, or weight loss surgery in particular. I'm only using them as examples. You can substitute any diet craze (eh-hem, program) and you will get the same results. This is why creating your own evidence-based program is essential.

When you are thinking about getting a pet or a new car you sort of have to ask yourself, "Am I a cat person? or a dog person? Or would I rather have a snake?" Or "How would I look in that bright red convertible... with all five of my kids?" You are constantly making these assessments about how well your choices fit with who you are. Maybe you need a minivan, but you get an SUV because you want to reflect a more sporty image and appear less like a 'typical soccer mom' - whatever that is. (When my kids were little I just wanted a car that was big enough that they couldn't touch each other!) Sometimes these choices are made almost unconsciously. You don't have to put a lot of thought into whether you want a cat or a dog because maybe you have always loved dogs.

But you can be more deliberate about some choices. And in order to become who you really want to be, you must be more deliberate about the related choices.

Another reason that diets have failed us in so many cases is that we have had the idea that all we have to do is to "get through" this cabbage eating phase of the diet, lose the weight, and the problem is gone. But we have already discovered that obesity is a life long disease that must be managed throughout your life. If you choose to manage it with cabbage, you must eat cabbage for the rest of your days.

Whatever you choose, you must be sure there are no flickers of doubt. If there is doubt, you must find a way to resolve that before it becomes mistrust. Once it becomes mistrust the diet is over, and you are back to square one or much much worse. The only way to be sure that you have no reason to doubt is to study what works for you. You will never have to wonder again if what you are doing is the right thing for you. The evidence is clear! Science does not lie. It is trustworthy and objective. It has no ulterior motives!

This stage is fundamental. By that I mean without successfully navigating this stage, the other stages are impossible. Unless you really understand your decisions regarding trusting any given lifestyle or program, you cannot begin to import that into your identity. We have just begun the process of identity development. There is much work to do.

This next thing is vital: Trust is not just based on your ability to trust.

You have proven over and over that you are able and willing to trust. The problem is that you've been trusting in all the wrong things.

Trust is also based upon the dependability and quality of your caregivers. In other words, if the diet program you choose is not completely dependable, your trust has been misplaced. I know a lot of well meaning, naive people who put their trust, and a lot of their available cash into 'reputable' diet programs with the hope that this could finally be the thing that cures their obesity. Unfortunately since 98% of all diets fail, we know our trust was misplaced 98% of the time. And now our money is gone too!

Here's the key to knowing you have successfully navigated this stage of identity development. When you are successful, you will have a sense of peace, safety, and satisfaction in what you are doing. If you haven't yet mastered this stage you may have feelings of fear, doubt, and a belief that the world is an unfair, inconsistent and unpredictable place.

Think about the times when you've tried so hard, worked your butt off literally, and the scale doesn't reflect that hard work. You don't feel like you should feel. Worse than that, you really feel like somewhere along the line your diet program has betrayed you! It's not logical! It's not predictable! It's happened to every serial dieter out there! And I consider myself one of the all time great serial dieters. You are not alone! It's not your fault. Stage One was not navigated successfully, and probably for good reason. Doubt became mistrust, and mistrust became an unpredictable, fear and anxiety producing experience. So you got out. Good for you! It wasn't right for you. Neither were any of the others. Neither was that rotten High School boyfriend. It's time to move on to what you can count on, what is right and authentically you. What does your authentically healthy life look like?

Take some time right now and write it down. Whatever came into your head just now, write that down. This is important.

How do you work through this stage successfully? Here are a few questions to help get you there. Be honest with yourself. Answer with reality in mind, not thinking about the best case scenario, or the diet guru's sales pitch. The important thing here is that your answers reflect your experiences. Think about your habits- the way you generally act and think. There are no right or wrong answers- only reality.

Write Your Story

Are your daily habits surrounding diet and movement the best you can do?

Is what you eat healthy? Honestly. Need some guidance in terms of what eating healthy means?

How often do you eat and drink only what is healthy for you? Daily? Weekly? When you're being watched? When you're reeling with guilt from a binge?

Would an alien race judge your diet and exercise habits as healthy for your specific body? (okay, that was just for fun)

Can you completely trust your diet and movement habits for the long term (until you are in your 90s)?

What do you think the outcomes of an autopsy on your body would be if it was done today? What about next year at this time (given your current diet and exercise habits)?

How do you feel about being associated with how you eat and move? (proud? a little embarrassed?)

Is there any guilt associated with how you eat or with your daily movement (or lack of)?

Are you embarrassed to eat in front of other people?

Are you proud of your exercise habits?

Do you talk about your exercise habits with other people who have similar routines?

Think about your last diet. How did you feel when it failed?

What about your last diet made you want to trust it before you started?

Where did the doubt about your last failed diet seep in?

Did you blame the diet program when it failed or did you blame yourself? Why?

What would your life look like if you never had to choose another diet again? How would that feel?

Do you think the world is a trustworthy place? Why or why not?

Is your diet predictable for the most part? Do you feel healthy and whole when you eat that way consistently?

Does your body react predictably to your diet? Can you predict your weight loss, your daily BMs, your energy levels, and your mood swings accurately?

Do you live in fear that if you "fell off the diet wagon" you would regain all your weight and then some?

After answering all these questions about your diet and exercise habits, sit back and take a look at what you have written. Now, take a deep breath and decide to make your last diet and exercise choice based on scientific evidence tailored specifically to your body's needs. Once you have determined your dietary needs, go back to the questions and answer them again, this time with your authentically healthy evidenced-based program in mind. This time answer them with the idea that you are going to become the authentically healthy person you have always wanted to be. Shed the neurotic, needy, navel-gazing, compulsive extremist behaviors that diet gurus count on. I think you will be amazed at what happens to your view of your life and your world!

Now exhale.

STAGE TWO: AUTONOMY

Toddlers must undergo one of the most challenging of tasks known to humankind: potty training. Okay, so maybe this is more challenging to parents than children. Seriously, I do think there is something monumental about this stage for the toddler. It is all about doing something brand new and succeeding at it. Potty training isn't for the faint of heart, and I sure would not want to have to do it as an adult! It is a very intimate, private, potentially humiliating event that nearly everyone must endure. Yet we tend not to be as sensitive about it as we could be. We make nervous jokes and congratulate the young one's successes, while we are secretly so glad we don't have to deal with diapers any more! I think it is easy to forget that this is potentially really difficult emotionally for the child.

After all, the toddler, through no choice of their own, has to change the way they are doing something they have done all their lives, and never look back. The toddler feels that what comes out of their little bodies is an extension of them! They literally think that their poo is part of them! They really identify with it! And it is only because of the intimate trust bond that you have formed with your little one that they even allow you to change their diaper in the first place! That, and they aren't coordinated or strong enough to stop you. <grin> Now you are asking them to part with the diapering experience and literally the poo in a way that is completely new to them! Flushing it can be really traumatic at first.

They must also say goodbye to the comfort of someone else taking care of them, and move to a place where they are taking care of themselves. That's harsh news to hear over your morning sippie cup.

No more diaper changes. Those times are being ripped from the child and they are being forced into something brand new. Sure, it is exciting! After all, there is UNDERWEAR! And everyone is so happy and congratulating you! But still, a little part of you misses the intimate times when someone else took care of you; without question they were there for you when you needed them. And at least at first you might have a crisis of confidence about going in a big potty! Could this be the right way to do it? It's SO different from what I am used to! But somehow you know it is going to be okay and that eventually it will become second nature to you.

After all, you've seen mommy and or daddy go this way. It must be ok. I trust them. I know them. And I want to be just like them! So, you go.

What could potty training possibly have in common with weight loss?! You might be surprised!

You began this journey learning that trust was absolute. You cannot move forward in your journey until you understand that the way you have done things in the past is childish and immature. Just like filling your diapers. You may have thought that as an adult you were doing the thing you had always done. It was comfortable, and in many ways it worked for you. It may even be based partly on some intimate, albeit childish relationships. But it wasn't healthy. And it wasn't the behavior of a mature, responsible adult.

In this analogy, your immature eating and exercise habits are like filling your diaper and waiting for someone else to come change them. You spent your life eating what you wanted to eat, or from time to time what someone else told you to eat. The fact that it wasn't healthy for you didn't cross your mind until you suffered some kind of consequence. Maybe that was obesity. Maybe that was high blood pressure. Many Americans subconsciously think that they can continue to eat an unhealthy, high calorie diet until someone else finally comes to rescue them from a heart attack! Never mind that the first symptom of heart disease is often death.

Truthfully, that's what so many of us look for in diet and exercise gurus. We want them to change our diaper! Take care of us. Tell us exactly what to do, taking the responsibility for potty training and independent responsible living out of our hands! If the diet guru can just tell us how to live, we can mimic them and they will take care of us. They will think for us. No need to think for yourself! Just do what they did, after all, it worked for them!

That, my friend is crazy. No, that is slavery. That is living life in a diaper!

The goal of growing up is to become an independent and responsible adult. It's that simple. That does not include depending upon some diet guru or personal trainer to the stars to change your diaper!

Let's look at the logical consequences of following one of these gurus. I don't have to spell it out for you. Just look back at the last few diets you attempted. When you finally fatigued so much from your attempts at white knuckling it, you crashed. The result was, as it always is, shame and self doubt.

It is important to note here that the reasons those diet gurus are successful is that they took responsibility for themselves, made their own choices, and moved to a place of maturity. But their choices are not yours. There is so much behind why their diet plan works for them, psychologically speaking, that you will possibly never know. Their journey is theirs alone, just as yours must be yours alone. They succeed because of the meaningful transitions that they have undertaken, but in the process of synthesizing that experience, boiling it down into a program, most of them have forgotten what it took for them to get there. (If indeed they were ever overweight to begin with!) Further, most of them are simply not well educated or insightful enough to see that you must progress through your own journey, just as they did, in order to succeed.

They expect you to simply apply the end results of their journey to your life. No process, no psychological work, just do what they did, and just like them you will be successful. "Eat cabbage soup" or "eat like a cave man" or "stop eating bread!" They exclaim from their mountain summit, "I did it, and look what it did for me!" Except you know from the tiny disclaimer at the bottom of the commercial that these results are not typical!

Understand this: YOU ARE TYPICAL. There's no shame in that. You are typical. In Western cultures, we don't like to think of ourselves as typical. For some of us that means we are not special. Many of us have it in our minds that no matter the odds, we can be the one person out of the hoards of people who will actually succeed. After all, that's the verbal message! You can do this! Shame on them for lying to us.

If you saw an ad that said, "take this medicine and if you are one of the lucky few, it will work for you! Two out of every one hundred people who take this medicine will get better! Two of you! Now, 98 of you will not get better, and you will probably have some nasty side effects too. But if you are super lucky, you could get better!" Would you be likely to jump on board with that new medication? I know I wouldn't! I would want to know that if I was going to risk having nasty side effects, that medicine would cure me!

If you are human, you are typical. You are part of the 98%! and just as surely as you needed to be potty trained, and you needed to move from being an infant to being a big kid, you need to create your own journey and stop expecting diet gurus to change your diaper!

The time has come for you to stop pretending to be someone you are not, and find out who you really are. It is time to stop mimicking the diets of others, and find out what works for you.

Through your own records and journals you will be able to study exactly what works for you. You will not only be able to see your progress, like in some online programs, but you will be able to run experiments that will result in more insight about what works for you, tweak it and run it again. In this way you will be creating your own, perfectly tailored program; not following the program of some guru. Experiment with what you know to be generally true, and not the exception to the rule. See how your body reacts. You can use the suggestions of others or begin with what you know about yourself and see what the data tell you. Act on the facts about you. Now you can know for certain what works for you. No more guess work or groundless hoping about the latest diet craze. I swear, I think that many people see a new diet ad and see one food in the ad (bacon or pizza) that they love and decide they can try the program based on that. Why not decide based on the facts. Not the facts about someone else. If you "love" bacon, test it! How does bacon effect you? Does it increase your energy? Help you lose weight? Or make your ankles swell? These are YOUR FACTS. That's worthy of committing to!

Now, for the next big issue: your emotions.

It seems to me that this is the part where on the reality TV show they say encouragingly, "you are going to need to work through those emotions!" Wow. It sounds good on the surface. But they are still not telling you HOW! How do I work through the anger I feel for being abandoned? Or abused? Or disrespected? How do I work through the years of self loathing based on the insensitive and mean-spirited comments from nasty relatives or strangers?

How do we face it all and put it into perspective?

One way to do that is by creating a new narrative. Your life is your story. We are a story telling people. We love stories. That's why TV and movies are so important to us! We communicate in stories. Think about it. You were late for work this morning, you rushed in drenched from head to toe, your umbrella is inside out, and your coffee has spilled all over your pants. Intuitively, we all know you have a story to tell! And we want you to tell it even though it is pretty clear from your appearance that you've been out in the wind and rain. We want you to tell your story because we want to share our (extremely similar) story with you! We do this as a way to share experiences that allow us to identify with and bond with one another. It would be completely unsatisfying if you came into the office like that with a completely emotionless expression and said nothing, gave no reaction, looked at no one, just went along with your day, wet pants and all. It might, depending upon your personality, cause the others in the office to giggle once you left the room. But they won't bond with you. They might bond with one another, but not with you. Your story is left to their imagination.

Whether you are a good story teller or not, your life is the most important story you will ever tell. Even if you are quiet, and prefer not to tell everyone you meet everything about you, you must find a way to tell your story. If all you do is to write it, you must tell it. Simply by living it, you are already telling it. Tell the story you want to tell. Tell your individual story.

THIS IS IMPORTANT. You are important. Your life is important. You are unique, and because you are unique your story must be told. Your voice should be heard, if even in writing and revealed only long after you have passed.

For some of us, the focus of our stories are those around us. We think that if we simply focus on our kids, grandkids, work, hobbies, etc. that is sufficient. By doing this, you are saying to the world that you are not important. You are saying that you have nothing to offer the world, and nothing to give. You are saying that your story is unimportant in the scope of the history of the world.

Nothing could be further from the truth and you know better than that. Even on your worst days in the middle of your best pity party, you know better than to think you are unimportant in the world.

So grow up and be willing to tell your story.

The first step in telling your story is also your first step in becoming a full fledged, responsible, individual, just as the first step in becoming a "big kid" was potty training. It is the first time in our lives when we stop being dependent on others and take responsibility for ourselves.

So, it is from this point on that you can look at yourself in the mirror and decide that you will be responsible for your life and for your own self care. It really is that simple. You must take care of yourself. What does that mean in practical terms?

It means that each day you get to make the choices that will result in becoming who you want to be. And as each choice is made, it brings your closer to becoming who you want to be. What you wear, what you eat, how you move, your smile, it all matters. If what you want is an authentic, integrated, healthy life, then choose to be real. Choose to eat what is real. Allow your healthy way of life to be reflected in all you do, what you wear, and who you associate with.

Make choices that are good for you. That's what taking care of yourself is all about. It might take some time to get the hang of it. No worries. You weren't perfect when you first began to potty train either! You slipped up, had accidents and made messes. But you continued on. You didn't give up and say, "to heck with this whole sitting on the toilet thing, I'm going back to diapers!" You might have wanted to, but you didn't. And you might have even had an overnight accident. Some situations are more difficult than others. That's okay! You still got through it.

I was always cheered when my kids were going through potty training by the thought that they were not going to be 40 years old wearing a diaper! And you will get through this transition too!

Here's the key: Autonomy. What does that mean? Autonomy is all about "self governing". You take responsibility for yourself, and you begin to govern yourself. You act in the best interest of your body and your mind. Do what you know is right for yourself. If you want to know for sure, test it. Experiment and know.

What if you've got a ton of emotional baggage? Most of us do. No one has lived a perfect life. Human interaction means we are all hurt from time to time.

So, take some time and write your story. First make a list of everything bad or painful that has ever happened to you. Then when you are satisfied that your list is complete take the first event on the list and write it out in as much detail as possible. Every feeling, every color, every person involved, name names, write the entire event in as much detail as you honestly remember. When you have finished writing the first event, take the second then the third, and write them all out.

Then when you've written every story, every bit of baggage you could possibly write about, take it and put it into an envelope. It might have to be one of those huge manila envelopes that you put the science project board into. But that's okay. On the outside of the envelope in huge letters write this: "Perspective"

You have now literally put all your baggage into perspective. Take a look around the room. Notice what's there. Your shoes, or a hat. Maybe there are some books on a table next to a mug. Now look back at your envelope. That's what having all those things in perspective is like. The envelope is just another item in the room of your life. It would be silly to let that run your life and make your decisions for you.

What does that mean and why is it important? The physical act of writing about the troubling events of our lives is therapeutic. For many of us writing these stories down means that we no longer have to hold onto them as object lessons that keep us safe. For some people the act of writing about difficult times in our lives gives us permission to stop living and reliving them. For some people writing simply allows us a safe place to let the emotions out. And no one has to read them.

For some of you, this may not be enough therapy. Some folks need more support to bring their stories out into the light. Some people need the unconditional positive regard that you can only get from a psychologist. Some people have so much pain that they need more than simply talking about their difficulties. Some of us need guidance and someone who will be there for us step-by-step. That's okay. In fact, you need to decide how much support you need in order to tell your story.

If you hate writing, get a cheap audio recorder and tell your story that way. You need to find a way that works for you. No excuses. Don't worry about grammar or spelling. It is not about how well you write or talk. It is about you processing the pain.

When you do this, you also take responsibility for who you have become and who you are becoming. And if you process through this, you won't ever choose to go back to wearing a diaper. You won't even want to! Being independent has a lot of perks! And you will never again need to imitate someone else's life, because you will be too excited about building your own!

Once you have done all that, move on to the next stage: Initiative versus Guilt.

STAGE THREE: INITIATIVE

This is the stage where I first realized that my choices in life were not enough to reinforce the changes I wanted to make in my life. This is the stage where the world pushes back. It is critical to understand this stage in order to progress and become who you really want to be. Of course all of these stages are important, but some of them are more intuitive than others. This, I believe, is one of the less intuitive, more difficult stages to understand. In other words, you may be faced with it and not even recognize what is happening to you, let alone react to it in a way that constitutes successfully navigating through it! Understanding stage three is a case where knowledge truly is power!

For as long as I have been dieting (probably 35 years) I have been under the impression that obesity is all about my choices. It's calories in, and calories out, right? If I have too much weight on my frame it is entirely my own fault. That's what we've been told for decades. No matter how many fads come and go, the diet industry always comes back to that. I have said many times, if dieting was just a physical problem we would have solved it ages ago. We all know that there is a psychological component to dieting that is just as important as the physical one.

So why is everyone so quick to dismiss and ignore it?

The reason boils down to the simple fact that when we honestly don't know what to do in a situation, we push it aside and ignore it. We hope that by focusing on the diet and exercise that the psychological stuff will somehow take care of itself! wow. Yup, that's been the hope for many decades now.

Obviously that is NOT HAPPENING! And it never will.

When Erik Erikson described this stage of human development, he noted that children come to a point in life when they realize that they have ideas about the world, and that they want to share them with others. They just aren't always sure of the best way to go about that. We've all met the kid who insists that if you swallowed your gum it would take 7 years for it to digest. It's only when the world, and hopefully reality, pushes back with just the right amount of pressure, that that kid finally stops insisting on his incorrect point of view. Or on the playground when the "bossy kid" starts pushing everyone into playing four square every day, eventually someone gets tired of four-square and pushes back. It's through these experiences that we learn just how much society will tolerate, even appreciate our ideas.

I remember a little girl on the grade school playground who was preaching salvation to all the first through third graders. She was preaching hell fire and brimstone and she wasn't taking prisoners. She and her posse would corner a kid in a remote part of the playground, convince them of their sin, and then scare them near to death with graphic stories of suffering and pain and hell. This got to be quite a problem when several of the children began having nightmares about going to hell. Eventually, the teacher got wind of the little girl's graphic and rather harsh techniques and pushed back. It was important for this little girl to learn that while she could share her beliefs with others, scaring them into believing was counter-productive. Once the teacher pushed back, that empowered the children to push back too, and to speak up when they had been cornered by the little evangelist. When she realized that her flock had turned against her and that her numbers were dwindling, she changed her tactics.

These kinds of interactions shape not only what we are willing share with others, but also how we see ourselves and our own ideas. If we happen to live in a repressed environment, it is likely we will grow up feeling our ideas are inferior or unworthy of being shared with others. And the converse is also true, if we grow up in an environment that never corrects us, kowtowing to our every whim, we are likely to believe that our ideas are infallible and we might have an over inflated sense of our value in relation to others.

When I was in the seventh grade I decided that class officer elections in my school were unfair and too exclusive. It seemed to me that nominations were limited to the rich and popular kids in class. So, I asked if I could enter the race myself. The teacher who was in charge of the whole thing was such an oaf that he literally laughed in my face and then made a joke of the idea in front of the entire class. And once they'd all had a good laugh at my expense, the teacher thought it would be doubly funny if he let me run for class president despite what a joke it was.

Mercifully, the whole election took less than five minutes. The teacher basically asked for a show of hands for each of the offices, leaving the office of president to last. When it came time to vote for class president he read out the name of the popular football captain and nearly every hand shot up. Then he read my name and just as quickly a roar of laughter rang through the room. I knew then and there what my place in that group would be for the next five years.

And I was right.

It is no coincidence that I began to gain weight that year for the first time and that I nearly failed the 7th grade. I felt ashamed of the fact that I had taken the initiative to right a perceived wrong.

How does this relate to weight loss maintenance?

I will answer that question by way of another story. When I had lost nearly 100 pounds after gastric bypass, my confidence was sky high. It was interesting that weight loss could afford me not only more confidence, but more opportunity too.

It's well documented that people who do not have obesity make more money and get more promotions and positions of higher authority than their equally qualified counterparts.

In any case, I was spreading my wings in my new position at work when out of the blue after less than a year in the position, I was fired! I'd never been fired in my entire life and although it was humiliating, it was the reason I was fired that really got my attention.

I was fired because the group I managed liked me better than they liked my boss. Before I took the position, my manager (we'll call him Dave) had been the Good Time Charlie of the office, the popular one. Despite the fact that Dave was a big phony-boloney (liar and scoundrel) he was the boss and as such he was the guy everyone kissed up to. Since there was no one else to turn to, everyone looked to Dave for answers and direction. Dave was happy in that role because despite the fact that his department was falling apart and unprofitable, he was popular, and that was all that mattered. He was a very shallow human being.

Then, at the behest of the board of directors, he hired me.

In no time at all people seemed to be drawn to me, as I was to them. I was told when I was hired that many things needed to change in my department, and that it would be up to me to change them. So I took the initiative and made sweeping changes. The creativity, productivity, and the morale of the group skyrocketed, and it didn't hurt the company's bottom line either! It took very little time before people who had previously looked to Dave, were looking to me, and that was appropriate. After all, I was their boss.

Unfortunately, this was a problem for Dave. He didn't like what had been happening. Despite the fact that he'd ordered me to make changes, he resented me and the changes I had made. He told me that I had taken too much initiative and that he'd liked things the way they had been for the last 14 years.

The morning he fired me he told me in no uncertain terms that he didn't like it that I was popular with the "grunts" (his word -

certainly not mine!). He said that he and I were too much alike, and that there could only be one of us in the company. Since he was part owner, it was obvious he wasn't leaving. He said that my new programs made him look bad to the board of directors, which happened to be his family. His family was disappointed that he had not thought of these ideas himself. And he told me that the longer I was there, the less valuable he looked to his family and to the company. So, he fired me.

I had taken initiative and the world, in the form of an egotistical, short sighted boss, pushed back. Needless to say I was devastated. Having never been fired before, I was humiliated. And because Dave had made it about me personally, by attacking my personality and my character during the firing process, I felt demeaned. It was Dave's goal to humiliate and disgrace me. He did a pretty good job of it too. For a long time I felt the strangest sensation of guilt. I couldn't figure out why I felt guilty. I had done nothing to merit guilty feelings. The meaning of this mystery would be revealed to me later.

Unfortunately, this was right at the time when I was diagnosed with Rheumatoid Arthritis and put on all kinds of medications like steroids and things like Cymbalta and Lyrica, that cause weight gain. It was one heck of a double whammy!

First, I was unable to figure out a way to bounce back from the devastation of being unfairly pushed out of doing a successful job. Then the physical stuff cascaded over me like an avalanche, leaving me buried and left for dead. I could no longer run the five miles a day I had been running. My body hurt so much that I spent most of my time in bed.

I can see now that failing to navigate stage three was one of the pivotal points in my weight regain. If the RA had struck in a better time frame, I would have been in a better place psychologically to handle it, to find alternatives for physical activity. But since I was swimming in self defeat, I was blind to the kind of proactive self care I needed.

In order to successfully navigate stage three you must both experiment with asserting yourself and after experiencing the inevitable push back, find a positive balance.

You must find a way to take initiative and to deal with the push back.

Whether you decide to take initiative in a more hospitable part of the world, where your ideas would be welcomed, or you change your message to better reflect the needs of your current audience; do the work. Take initiative somewhere. Track it and see what works for you. You no longer have to guess! The science has been done, all you must do is apply it to your situation. Take advantage of the crowdsourcing information gathered from people across the world. These online tracking programs work as well on psychological processes as they do to determine your best diet or exercise program.

However if you fail, as I did, to navigate this stage successfully you will find yourself dogged by undeserved guilt. You will suffer shame and you may even be confused by it the way I was. I was ashamed of myself for sticking my neck out. I was ashamed that my efforts hadn't been appreciated, in either my job or my attempts to make the seventh grade class elections more democratic.

Many people who have spent the majority of their lives dealing with the disease of obesity have issues with self confidence. We have been shot down so many times that many of us withdraw from positions of leadership, and from speaking our minds in public just to avoid the possibility of painful push back.

But you must learn to deal with push back in a positive way in order to travel through this stage successfully. The first thing to realize is that push back isn't always right or justified. Just because some one decides your initiative isn't welcome, that doesn't give them a license to stop you.

There are lots of reasons people "push back" at you. Many of those reasons are selfish and have little or nothing to do with you at all. People will push back because they perceive that you are taking some of their power or in "Dave's" case their popularity. My 7th grade teacher was more concerned with being popular with the kids in my class than in conducting fair class elections. That did not make my initiative less important or my assertion that the election was rigged any less true. But the teacher held all the power and he pushed back with it. And I let him push me into silence.

I have been very careful since those times about making assertions and taking initiative. I find that if I am going to make an assertion, I want it to be grounded in facts and based in research. It is one way that I have found to mediate the effects of people who push back. This way, when I make an assertion and people push back, I am willing to counter push because I know what I am saying is based in evidence. I have learned to trust myself and my own opinions in this way.

I have determined that the balance is to take what others say seriously, weighing it against what I know. If what they say has more validity than my assertion, I will consider changing my thinking. However, if their assertions are based in selfishness and unfounded assumptions rather than facts, I am now able to put it behind me. It does not matter how powerful the person is, or how loudly they talk or how forcefully they make their points. It doesn't even matter that they might attempt to humiliate me in public as a way to push back.

Looking back I feel kind of silly about feeling guilty about interrupting the class elections to make a point. I wish I had not allowed my teacher to humiliate me in front of the class. I feel a bit silly about how long it took me to realize that I felt guilty about doing a good job and for being a popular leader in my job. I had nothing to feel guilty about. I should have felt pride, the way I do now when I think about those situations. I am proud of myself for standing up for clean and fair class elections, especially when none of my friends would stand with me. I am proud of the job I did in my position in Dave's company. I breathed life into a dying, stale organization. Where there was once shame and humiliation, there is now pride and self-confidence.

Remember when the world pushes back at you, the pushers are not automatically right. No matter who they are. Remember that you must take initiative, and learn to deal effectively with push back, in order to show the world who you really are. Remember that you belong as much as any one else in the world.

Remember that your opinions are valuable. And most of all, remember that in many cases you can and should push back, when you need to assert yourself and face the challenges in your path. You will want to pick your battles wisely. But when something is important to you, push back. It is that kind of give and take with the world that allows you to find your place in it.

Navigating this stage successfully means finding a place of self-confidence, where your initiative is valued, if only by yourself.

The choices you make for your diet and exercise are vital. Unfortunately they are not enough. You must also contend with the world around you. You live with and around people. Your choices effect not only you, some of your choices effect them too. Realizing that the world will push back, that there are others who do not share your passion for health and for being real, is the next step in your journey. It is why this is not just a psychological theory, but also a social theory too. That's why it is called a psycho-social theory. It has to do with you and the social world you live in.

In terms of long term health related lifestyle decisions, you must take initiative. You must be confident enough in the lifestyle you have chosen (have absolute trust) to be able to stand up to those who would push back against it. Know that your choices are good ones, and be able to defend against those whose motives are not in your best interest. You are building your authentically healthy life. Don't let anyone rob you of that, even if it seems at first to infringe on or disrupt their right to be unhealthy.

My husband has said for many years that when you do what is right for you, it will be right for everyone around you too. It may not seem like that at first. It might seem like stopping some of your unhealthy habits will hurt your relationships with the people who share those habits with you. For example, if you quit smoking, you may no longer take the time to visit with your smoking friends outside the back door at work. You may have to find other ways to interact with the people you want in your life. Rather than avoiding game night because it is difficult for you not to eat junk food, maybe you may need to assert yourself and change the food options available at game night. Maybe you should take the initiative and suggest more physically active games.

Unfortunately, I've spent a great deal of my adult life looking for a place that "wanted and accepted" me. I see now that was a mistake. That is a child's attitude. I now see the world differently, as an adult. Instead of looking for groups who would accept me or a place where I belong, I am focused on creating and building my own life. The life I want to live. If people want to fit with me, they simply become part of my life.

I am a part of the lives of others. But after navigating this stage I see that differently too. I no longer crave their approval. I no longer feel desperate for others to accept me. The amazing and paradoxical thing about this is that while I was a child in my thinking I felt very alone and isolated socially. Now my life is filled with people and social interactions that are healthy and I work toward more balanced alone time. The isolation is gone!

Push back can come in many forms. It is important that you see and understand that. It may come in a straightforward manner, like the examples above. Or it might come in more subtle forms, like your Ex consistently messing up your exercise schedule by not picking up the kids when it is his turn. My friend Micki shared a brilliant insight about push back with me this morning. She wrote this to me in an email: "I was thinking about the concept of "pushback" and how it may relate to women who have been sexually abused or raped; since there is often a reluctance to look "attractive" and a feeling of protection afforded by extra weight; hence the pushback may be strongly generated from within." We can generate our own push back as a protective measure!

However it comes, recognize it for what it is. Stay focused and look for solutions to problems that stand in your way. Reinvent, be creative but continue to work toward building your place. If you don't you could end up regaining your weight and missing out on living your healthy, authentic life.

Write Your Story

Think of times in your life when you experienced push back that stifled you. Write about times when you had lost weight, increased your confidence and took initiative. What kinds of push back did you experience? Who pushed back?

Write about why it is significant to think about who is doing the push back.

Write about ways you can creatively take initiative in ways you know you can and should.

How can you build your place in society? What do you want your place in society to be?
Write about how taking initiative can help get you there.

What would happen if you took initiative and got severe push back? How would you cope with that? How would you get around it?

Write about the life you want to build for yourself. What do you want to focus your days on? How will you use initiative to build a healthy authentic life that is consistent and productive?

If you are in a situation where you are unsure of how to proceed, experiment with it. Keep track online and find out what behavior gets you the results you want and what doesn't. Taking initiative can be done in many ways. See which one gets you the furthest toward your goal with the least amount of push back.

I would love to read your stories; both your successes and your challenges. I think that sharing these things can help us move through the stages. If you want to share them, contact me. I'd love to hear from you! Email me at carrieon@mac.com

STAGE FOUR: PRODUCTIVITY

This stage holds the key to true maturity. Are you a producer? Or are you a consumer? When you are a consumer, you do just that. You spend all your time, brain power and effort on consuming in one way or another. As someone who suffers from the complexities of obesity, you are focused on consuming in either a direct or indirect way, all day, every day.

Let me explain by way of showing you our ongoing connection to childhood. Children are consumers. It's all we know when we are born. We consume to survive. Without being focused on that, we would all die. It is a necessity for life... for babies.

You understand the concept of "net income" right? That's the amount of income you have left over when you've taken out taxes and paid your bills and met other responsibilities. We will apply the same concept to finding out how to become a net producer. When you truly mature you become a net producer. What that means is that you simply produce more than you consume. It is the only way to get ahead. It is true in finance and it is true in matters of health.

What I mean when I am talking about producing may not be entirely intuitive. What producing involves is the act of being productive. In order to tell whether you are a net producer or a net consumer in this world you really need to take stock and think about what you do, hour by hour, all day long. What activities are you involved with that produce a positive effect in your life or the lives of others?

Let me just say that while everyone needs rest, watching TV or movies is not being productive. And it isn't actually the most restful thing you could do! Most people get that, yet we watch a tremendous amount of television and movies. We consume hour after hour of entertainment like Facebook, video games, youtube, and mindless internet surfing. Consuming entertainment is not productive. But keep in mind, there are many forms consuming can take, including spending money. If you shop to drive the blues away, you might want to rethink your strategy. It is pure consumption and consuming is a childish activity. It is no way to deal with pain. Chances are that it doesn't work for long anyway, if in fact it works at all.

That's not to say that you've got to give up every indulgence to be healthy. But remember, you have a disease and this disease needs constant, vigilant treatment. The treatment must be consistent, because if it isn't, you will become sick. It's just like any other disease that way. So, day by day, in fact, hour by hour, these things matter. Each day that you are a net consumer (define consumer in the widest possible terms) you are functioning as a person who is a slave to your childish nature.

Each day that you produce more than you consume is a day when you have taken another step toward being the person you want to be: mature, healthy, integrated, whole, and authentic.

If you are a child, or act like a child in this regard, you will consume at will. Each whim is answered with 'yes'. You are indulging your childish nature with each treat. You are consuming to satisfy your childish desires, or to stop you from experiencing difficult emotions.

Think about it as if there is a child inside you. When you want that piece of cake, or those fries, or that second helping, think about the child inside you. What would you say to a child who constantly wants things that are not good for them? I think of the kid who is forever begging for what they want, tugging incessantly on my shirt sleeve. Of course you would not give them everything they desire! When you do, you know what happens. That child learns that all it takes to get their way is to tug at your sleeve. The more you indulge the child within, the more the child within will demand. Refuse the child things that are bad for you, and you will eventually learn that what is good for you is what you want anyway.

It comes down to two things. Self discipline and an acquired taste. Since everything is an acquired taste, it is logical to assume that if you choose the good stuff, eventually you will truly enjoy it. Maybe sooner than you think! Self discipline is harder to come by. Our society does not teach us self discipline. This is something that we must seek to learn on our own. That's tough to do!

The child inside you is the disease of obesity talking to you. Obesity IS the child. When my kids were little and would complain about having to eat healthy foods I would explain to them that I had to make their food choices for them until they were mature enough to make those good choices themselves. If my kids had their way they would have eaten jellybeans all day long... until they got sick.

A whole lot of folks have eaten boatloads of metaphoric jellybeans their whole lives and now they are sick. No big surprise there!

If you have obesity, it is probably largely due to the fact that you have been giving in to that kid inside you for years! You want something, and instead of being self disciplined and doing what you know is right, you give in. Over and over you give the child the treat to quiet the crying, or to make them happier, or to keep them from boredom. Sometimes the child inside simply doesn't want to put out the effort, so you choose what is easily available. You name it. There are as many reasons to give into that child inside you, as there are people. There is only one real reason not to give in to the child inside you: good health. And it is the most important thing in your life.

Children are also typically short sighted. They want immediate gratification and they aren't thinking about the long term effects of their choices. For children the long term can be as short as the tummy ache they will get after too many jellybeans. Many of them can't think even that far into the future. And many don't learn from the mistake of doing it once. They will continue to make that same mistake whenever there are jellybeans available.

I hope by now you can see yourself in this analogy. I know I have done it a hundred times! I have overeaten or eaten the thing that made me feel bad (physically or emotionally or both), even though the last three times it happened the result was the same. That is us being controlled by an out of control spoiled child. There is no way we would treat an actual child like that! We would never give in to them like we give into our inner child. Maybe once in a while, but not every single day the way many of us choose to live, giving into our inner child.

Part of the reason we give in has to do with a lack of balance in our lives. We don't get enough rest, nutrition, love, exercise, sunlight, etc. and as a result we live our lives day after day, feeling deprived. So we consume in order to attempt to fill those needs. But just like a lot of life, this is a paradox. The paradox is that what we need more than anything is to be productive.

Emotion is really complex. That's why there are people like me who spend a great deal of their lives studying psychology. These are not easy issues, but if you can approach these whims and desires with the child inside you in mind, you might be able to begin to separate yourself from those choices.

Why is it important to separate yourself from your choices? It's important because it is the only way to be objective about the things you choose. We have discovered that it is common for us to tie our identity to our jobs, for example. It is just as common to tie our identity to our choices. "I'm a non-fat double shot coffee person" or "I love ice cream" or "I'm vegan". If we can choose to see the most difficult part of this whole process (emotional eating) as separate from our identity, it gives us a fighting chance to become less a consumer and more a producer.

Further, being productive can in many many cases keep us from being focused on consuming. It really is an "either-or" proposition.

I can't count the number of times I have heard someone complain about the new diet they were on saying, "I hate it that I am focused so much on food! It is all I think about now!" I have experienced the same thing! I was so focused on food, weighing, measuring, counting each calorie, that I had little time to do or think about anything else! At first, it was kind of fun and even exciting to try to see how well I could do, watching the scale for progress. Each day that passed I would do a little better, cook a new low fat version of something, maybe get more fiber, less fat. It was kind of a game in the beginning. But inevitably there would come a day when I could no longer focus on how many celery sticks I had eaten. I no longer cared! And I wanted to think about something else! I had a life before I started the diet, and little by little that life was showing up and demanding that I get back to focusing on it. Further, I wanted to get back to my life! I had things I wanted to do with my life that did not involve weighing a piece of salmon! It is just that simple!

What I was craving was productivity! I wanted to do something productive with my life, not just focus on what I was consuming. Yes, it is important that you are selective about what you are consuming. It is also important that you do not stop consuming. That's anorexia. That's why I approach the goal in this stage as being a "net producing" lifestyle. It is all about finding the positive balance.

Think about your life today. What have you done today that involved consuming and what have you done that involved producing? This week, maybe even this month, keep a journal of your activities. Make a note next to each activity that you are involved with and categorize it as either a "productive" or "consuming" activity. At the end of each day or week, count the time you have spent producing and the time you spent in consuming activities. Take the number of hours you spend producing and subtract the number of hours you spent consuming, preparing to consume, or thinking about consuming. Count anything you do that involves creating something, learning something, discovering something, answering a need (like organizing your closet for example), activities with loved ones or to better yourself in some way, as productive behavior. Count anything that involves giving into your inner child, eating, shopping, watching, anything passive, as consuming behavior.

The idea here is to increase your productivity while decreasing your psychological need for consuming things you don't need. Why is this important? It is important for our sense of self confidence. If we fail to do this, the result is inferiority. We will feel inferior to others around us. When we are net consumers, we are not industrious. We are, in fact, mental children. We see ourselves as less than others. We cannot be whole as net consumers because in order to be whole we must grow up. We must be mature. We must mature the child within us to the point where they intuitively want to make good choices. In fact the maturing child within us should eventually mesh psychologically with our outer adult. That is integrity. Don't think too literally about this. It is a metaphor. But I think it is apt and it is one way to understand this stage and how to navigate through it successfully.

So the next time your inner child wants that frozen Snicker's bar, step back from the freezer and think about what's best for you in the long term. What will you teach your inner child? Will you give in and teach the child that whatever they want is ok with you? Remember in that moment that you have a disease. If you have Type One Diabetes, you would not "give in" to your inner child who doesn't want to take her insulin shot! That could kill you! Remember, this disease, if left untreated will continue to make you sicker and sicker. If it continues to progress, it will kill you. In the mean time, you will not live an authentic, whole and healthy life. You will be of two minds: your adult mind who knows what choices you should make, and your inner child's mind who wants jellybeans for every meal.

Like self esteem, self confidence comes not from telling yourself how great you are, but from accomplishing something difficult. This is truly difficult. Build your self confidence and you will master this stage and be that much closer to who you want to be. It is going to take some work, but I promise you it is worth it in so many ways.

Write Your Story

Write about three consumer behaviors (not including eating) that you would like to change and how you plan to change them.

How can these changes enrich your life? Will they?

Once you have made these changes go back and write about how your life was and how it is after the changes.

STAGE FIVE IDENTITY

What we look like to others is of some importance to most of us. But do we really know how others see us? And does the person they see jive with the person we want to be? Most of us have had the experience of hearing our own voice on an audio recording. The experience is most often followed by the common, incredulous reaction, "Is THAT what I sound like to you?!" And I am still surprised when the answer is yes. I sound so different inside my head.

The same is true in terms of how I look in the eyes of others, but to varying degrees. My children (like most kids) don't see me in physical terms. They see me as "Mom" in the same way that I don't see my own mother in physical terms. But most people we encounter during the course of the day see us primarily as our physical representation, especially if they do not know us well.

Those who know us best are often able to look past what is familiar to the core of who we are. Sometimes that is a real advantage, sometimes it is a detriment. It is one of the reasons couples gain weight together. They stop noticing one another physically, in a sense. That doesn't mean their attraction for one another necessarily dies. It might mean that. But it probably means that the levels at which you are attracted to one another run much deeper than the physical. That is a good thing. Being truly known for who you really are is a precious commodity. But it can be a detriment for us in terms of promoting health behaviors and authenticity.

One of the biggest things to know about authenticity is that being authentic means to be in alignment. It means that what you believe is what you say. It means that what is important to you is reflected in what you do. It also means that what is on the inside should eventually be reflected on the outside as much as possible. I understand there are limits for some of us. I will never be six feet tall no matter how much I want to be. I am basically shaped like a hobbit. I come from a long line of hobbit like people, and it is part of my genetic reality. Some parts of that I can change by choice (hairy feet for example) but height is just not something we know how to change yet. Maybe some day. Until then, I am content with the aspects of my personage that I cannot change, and happy to change for the better where I can.

Let me be clear. This is a life long pursuit for most of us. And obesity, like any disease, can make it really difficult to bring the body into alignment with our minds and our beliefs and our values. It's the same as if you had cancer. The disease has a profound impact on your body. You may gain weight, you may lose weight, your skin may not glow the way it did when you were a child. All diseases have an impact on the body that is readily seen by those around us. And no matter what the disease, the fact that you have a disease makes it a lot harder to be seen for who you really are. It can take longer to look past a wheel chair or severe obesity, for example, when first getting to know someone.

It is well understood that people who suffer from obesity also suffer stereotypes and prejudices. The more of us afflicted with this complex disease, the more we see and understand the prejudices. You might think that since in America over 60% of us have obesity that we would represent a majority and that prejudice would simply fade away. The problem is that even those with the disease of obesity are prejudice against others with obesity! True! We may be more prejudiced than our healthier brothers and sisters in this regard. Part of the reason for that is that we are reflecting our own self-disappointment. Part of that is a direct reflection on how harshly we judge ourselves. It is important for you to understand this issue, from a human rights perspective. More on that when we do the exercises at the end of the chapter.

Your identity is really all you have when it comes down to the final assessment. Who you are is all you have. Whether you believe in some particular religion or philosophy, or none at all is immaterial. In the end what you have is who you have been throughout your life. That must be integrated with those beliefs, philosophies, or religious tenets.

It is important then to work on who you are and to be deliberately who you want to be. So many of us leave this to chance or our daily whims. We sort of become the sum of our experiences and many of us live a reactionary life. By that I mean that we go through life simply reacting to the events that happen around us, putting out metaphorical fires as they flare up. And in a survival based existence that might have been good enough. If all your energy is spent struggling to survive while you travel across America in a covered wagon, hoping to settle the untamed lands west of civilization, you probably don't have a problem with obesity. In fact, obesity rates were very low in the early days of America among people who colonized the western part of our country. Obesity is a disease of opportunity that thrives in times of plenty.

For those folks it was enough to live a reactive life. There was a lot to react to! But modern convenience, technology and progress have removed most of the difficulties of mere survival.

Erikson coined the term "identity crisis" to identify the transition we go through from childhood to adulthood. In fact, as we grow up we develop many identities. We are mothers or fathers, sisters or brothers, friends, class clowns, serious musicians, role models, bosses, employees, and the list goes on and on. Many of those identities are ones we are born into, or that we happen into through our different experiences. And these roles are all important to differing degrees. It is in these different positions that we allow others to see us as simply a part of that role. If I am a manager, then I leave the company and stay connected to some of my employees, it takes a concerted effort to change the dynamic in our relationship. Sometimes it doesn't work to change the dynamic, depending upon how long you have played those roles. It takes living a deliberate life to make changes like that.

Sometimes we find it difficult to step away from the roles we play in order to work on our most important role: our authentic self. You must be deliberate in your efforts to change from who you have been to the person you want to be. Health behaviors are no different. Health or ill health is a big part of our identity.

But when it comes to our health, many of us feel we are born into what we have. To some degree that is true. We have inherited a certain body type, a DNA sequence that determines our susceptibility to certain diseases, and even birth defects. But within those inherited traits choices still remain. We still possess a free will, and the freedom of choice to be who we really want to be, act in a manner we admire and respect, believe what we want. No matter your genetic heritage, you can choose who you will be.

How do we choose when so much of life is thrown at us at the speed of a bullet train? It is precisely in those times that our conscious choices mean the most. Those times are the tests. If your life is one endless string of activities at the speed of a bullet train, you might want to slow it down for a time while you go through this process. In order to live a deliberate life you must be able to breathe, take in some silence, rest an appropriate amount. Life at the speed of sound doesn't leave room for being deliberate.

I see families rushing from activity to activity, day in and evening out. Children up at 4 or 5 in the morning to get ready for sports practices and involved in activities late into the evening every single night. That's an extreme, but it is far more common than I wish it was. In those scenarios even if you are super organized and can keep all those balls in the air, including maintaining a home, timely haircuts and dental appointments for everyone, and priorities at work, it still doesn't leave much time for self- reflection and healthy personal growth, let alone eating right and exercising.

At some point in a world so rushed, something is bound to break. The American divorce rate would suggest that often it is our most intimate relationships that suffer. American obesity rates indicate to me that for most of us our health suffers greatly on the altar of a busy life.

Why are we so busy? It is a combination of things. I think that part of it is that busy-ness can mimic a full and satisfying life. It might be full, but it isn't always satisfying. Part of it is that some of us deliberately become busy to avoid dealing with tough emotional issues. Some of us plan an over abundance of public family time in order to avoid intimate family time. Some of us simply have no real identity of our own, so we fill our lives with so many roles in hopes of finding one that fits us. It brings to mind the saying: 'Throw enough spaghetti at the wall some of it is bound to stick". But that's not living deliberately or authentically.

In order to live a truly full and satisfying life, you must be deliberate about working toward your authentic self. Being who you want to be in every way, merging your thinking with your choices and with your image is all a part of that.

What does all of this have to do with weight loss? In order to eat deliberately you must make choices that are deliberate. For example, when you are hungry do you grab a handful of chips? or do you cut an apple and eat it with a little peanut butter? More fundamentally to our culture, do you go through the drive-thru or do you prepare meals from scratch? I know families who pick up drive -thru meals on their way home after their activities and serve fast food on plates at home as if they had cooked it themselves. Restaurant food used to be reserved for birthdays, anniversaries or other special days, and has now become a steady diet for a lot of people! And most restaurants are in the business for profit, not for your health.

When profit is involved, the first thing that suffers is your health. Restaurant food is not the same as what you would make at home, no matter how the ads read. Restaurants use the same 3 or 4 food manufacturers who distribute the same basic ingredients all across the country. It is the only way restaurants make a profit. Their margins are often so thin that they must use these "food-like" products in place of healthy, real food just to stay in business. They replace chicken with MSG, they use far too much salt, fat and sugar just to make sure your taste buds are fooled by the "food-like substances" they are serving you. Trans Fats still are commonplace in many restaurants. Fresh ingredients are rarely used without heavy preservatives. Witness the salad bar with its many preservatives! It takes a lot of chemicals to keep those greens looking good all day! Vegetables are often so overcooked as to be of little nutritional value, assuming you can get a vegetable in a restaurant these days! Of course I am not counting ketchup and fries. It is no mystery why as Americans eat out more and more often, we get sicker and sicker with each passing year. We are paying a heavy price for convenience, and even if you reserve eating out for celebrations, which some families still do, it is kind of a perverse thing to do. We are celebrating someone's life or accomplishments by getting the whole family together to literally inflict pain on our bodies. Perverse. (for details click here for more about this in- chapter 8)

One of the biggest reasons cited for not exercising is a lack of time. But those same folks who simply do not have time to exercise (or to cook, by the way) still have Facebook accounts, their favorite television shows, eating in restaurants (which generally takes a lot longer than eating at home) all kinds of gadgets that suck up tons more time than what it would take to get real exercise. The perception that we don't have time to work out has more to do with not being deliberate about our choices, and in not being deliberate we inadvertently choose to live a reactive life. We are already too busy (doing things that don't contribute to our health) to fit one more thing into our busy lives. If that is the case, your busy life will likely be synonymous with a short life. If you do not take care of your body, you will not live as long as you could have. It's that simple.

So the answer is pretty easy. Prioritize and plan. Drop something that you are doing, and be deliberate with your time. It might mean that you simply adjust how you are using that activity. You could walk on your treadmill while you watch your favorite show. This may keep you from snacking while you watch. Snacking while watching is a bigger problem than just watching TV!

Fidelity is key in this stage. Once you have passed through the previous stages, decided to be a producer rather than a consumer, built your own autonomy and initiative, you must next consider fidelity. This stage is crucial because fidelity means to sustain the promises to yourself (and to others) despite the possible contradictions that you may encounter.

All too often we are moving ahead in our diet and exercise program when we come across something that contradicts the core ideas of what we are doing! It is inevitable in this culture of pop-up dieting where there is a new diet crazy in the media nearly every day! Seriously, you need only to turn on the television one afternoon to see what I am talking about! And these are not all "fly by night" diet gurus! Most of them are trusted doctors! It is so easy to jump from diet to diet, hoping the latest one brings you more success than the last! But remember this: you have finally taken the necessary time, energy and thought about what you have chosen to align yourself with in terms of the way you eat, the kind of exercise you get and what that means for your new identity.

This is something new for most of us! It's probably the first time you have spent considerable time and given an ample amount of reflection before making diet and exercise decisions. Get used to the idea that this is a process through which you are fundamentally changing who you are in order to build (re-build) your identity. This is about living a deliberate life.

So, during this stage be mindful that the instinct to jump ship and try something else that's new, is common. You aren't alone. You may never have been as aware before now that you have been doing this. And some of what's out there isn't bad. If you can incorporate it into your new identity, and it helps you reach your goals, go for it. But be mindful of the pledges you have made to yourself in the past that you have broken. Today's new diet idea might just be another distraction.

What's important is that you are mindful that the choices you make in this process will either push you toward success and long term weight loss or they will hinder your long term success. What do you want your outcome to be? Think long term when making daily decisions and you will have long term success.

What do you want your image to be? Do you want to be seen by others as flying from activity to activity, diet to diet, Jack of All Trades, Master of none? Or do you want to be deliberate in your choices and own your image? Do you want to be someone who jumps from one diet fad to the next? Or do you want to be seen as someone who knows their own mind? Do you want to be seen as a couch potato? Or as someone who is healthy and vibrant? You can't be both. And no matter how symptom free you are today, your couch potato lifestyle will catch up with your genetics. So you have a choice. You can be in control of your own destiny, living a deliberate life, or you can roll with what life throws at you, running from fire to fire, never moving ahead with your personal goals and never becoming the person you really want to be.

You can be confused about who you are, or understand and

deliberately develop who you want to be. How does it look to be confused about who you are? Your lifestyle changes with the winds. You allow others to make choices that affect your time and energy. You see yourself as dramatically different from how others see you. Those are the symptoms of role confusion. Self confidence, on the other hand, is the outcome of a well developed and thoroughly thought out identity. Health and vibrancy are the hallmarks of a life well lived. Undoubtedly you have experimented with all kinds of identities and roles for yourself. It is time now to chose to be healthy, balanced, and authentic.

Time to Write

Write out all the roles you play in your life.

What roles suit you best?

What roles are counterproductive to your goal of getting and staying healthy?

Is there any way to change the counterproductive parts of your life? Really give this some creative thought. If you need some ideas, we are online and the community might have some wisdom for you on this!

What roles conflict with who you want to be? What will you do about that?

1. Write a list of words that describe your self image.

2. Now write a list of words that represent how others see you? You might have to really think about this. Look in the mirror with this question in mind.

3. Write a list of words that represents your ideal self image?
Now see if there are any commonalities between the last two lists.

What's different?

What would you like to be different?

What can you do to make list #1 & #2 contain more items from list #3? Think in concrete, actionable terms. For example, if I want to be seen as more knowledgeable about books #3 might contain a list of books I will read to be more well read, and a speed reading course I can take online for free. Put some thought into these. And don't limit them to diet and exercise goals. Not everyone can be a personal trainer. But if that's what you love, put it on the list! This is your image we're sculpting!

STAGE SIX: INTIMACY

As you solidify your identity as a healthy authentic person, it becomes apparent very quickly that there are some people in your circles, maybe even your inner circles, who are not in alignment with your goals. How do we maintain our new identity in the real world? Be careful Dear Ones, that those with whom you merge are good for you. We tend to become like those we spend the most time with. Therefore you should choose friends and partners who have high standards and values that you espouse. You have to think about that when you consider your relationships. Is this someone I want to be more like? Are they active? Healthy? Consistent? Do not fool yourself into thinking that they will become more like you and that you will remain the same. It almost never happens that way. We all affect one another in big and small ways when we interact and we inadvertently become like those we spend time with.

It is not impossible to successfully blend your new identity with those who are important to you. It depends to some extent how healthy they are, and their attitudes about the changes you are making in your life. If they are stubbornly unhealthy, it might be difficult to maintain your new identity while remaining intimate with someone who is unhealthy and unwilling to change. But I think that is the exception to the rule.

This of it like this: you are kneeling on top of a very high table. Your partner is on the floor but just within your reach. You clasp hands and each person begins to pull the other one toward them. What will certainly happen? The person on the floor will pull the person on the table down to their level. Gravity dictates this. It isn't for lack of trying that you topple to the floor. It is simply physics. The same is true in terms of living a healthy life. If you attempt to pull an unwilling partner up to your level, you may be able to struggle with them for a time, but inevitably, they will pull you down into their unhealthy lifestyle. After all, let's face it. Being unhealthy is much easier than being healthy.

Many of you have already "merged" your lives with others who are not good for you. It happens frequently to people who suffer obesity. Many people allow obesity to lower their self confidence and they settle for mates who are not focused on their best interests. It is a common and sad story. Some even put up with abuse because the fear of being alone is stronger for them than the harm produced by the physical and emotional pain. There are a lot of reasons for this.

Intimacy is tricky.

You need to maintain who you are, who you are becoming, and at the same time, form intimate relationships with others.

Here's the test: When you are with your significant other are you able to be fully authentic?

It is impossible to make the sacrifices necessary to a healthy relationship, if while you are in the relationship you are not able to be authentic.

While we all wear slightly different hats with different people we know, the intimate relationships we have must be the ones in which you can be completely yourself. If that isn't the case, it may be time to reevaluate.

Why is this important? It's vital because your goals and dreams and state of physical and emotional health are the cornerstone of your experience in this world. If there is a difference in world views between you are a significant other, you will choose to be loyal to yourself, or to the other. You may be able to agree to disagree about certain healthy behaviors. In this way it is possible to merge your health goals with someone else, as long as they value you as a person, and want the best for you in this life.

I heard someone respond to this point with, "My relationship with my husband is more important to me than exercising!" What that tells me is that this person prizes her husband over her health. She does not care for herself in the way she should. Further, I would bet that her husband does not care about her long term health or even his own. You must first put on your own oxygen mask, in order to help anyone else. In other words, you must care about your own health first and foremost, before anyone or anything else. That includes significant others. You must care about yourself first and foremost.

This might sound completely selfish, but it isn't. I've heard psychologist Dr. Phil McGraw say that one of his fondest wishes is that people would stop thinking that taking care of themselves is selfish.

It is simply you taking care of what was entrusted to you at birth. We value people in our culture who take care of everyone around them. Unfortunately, they most often do that at the risk of neglecting themselves. Self sacrifice in this sense is not a healthy behavior. If you are so busy taking care of all those around you that you neglect yourself you are not really taking care of them. You are teaching them to be dependent upon you, which is unhealthy for both you and them.

Further, you are teaching the next generation that we do not value taking care of ourselves. This problem, in our culture, most often falls to mothers and women in general, although I have known men who suffer from this kind of shortsightedness too.

Women are nurturers by nature. We know that nurturing has been a behavior that has kept us as a species alive over centuries of harsh environments that threaten the lives of our offspring. And despite the changes in our environment, there is still a place for nurturing behavior. No doubt about it. But understand your own goals and the goals you have for your family. If your goals for your children include raising healthy, independent and responsible adults, too much nurturing will not get you there.

Children do not learn what we tell them. They learn from our behaviors. So all the yelling and begging and lecturing in the world will not sink in if your actions contradict your words. This is important. The reason it is vital is in understanding what it means to be authentic. When your behavior and speech match, you are more likely to have an impact on your family's behaviors. If you want to teach your children to take care of themselves, take care of yourself. If you take care of them at the expense of your own health, you can expect that when they become adults taking care of themselves will not be a priority.

Sometimes in families with both sons and daughters, sons will be taken care of while daughters are taught skills like cooking and laundry. In Italy part of their culture includes single men living at home into their 30s and beyond to make it convenient for their mothers to take care of them. They treat it like it is an act of mercy to move in (or continue into adulthood) with their parents so that mom doesn't have to lug her son's clean laundry across town. Now I am all for cultural diversity and appreciation. But that seems like one symptom of pretty big problem.

You might be lucky enough to have a partner who is healthy in mind and body, who also cares about your health and wellbeing. I sincerely hope that is the case. But if it is not the case, you cannot even hope to change that person until your change is solid and complete. Until you are healthy you can have no long term or lasting effect on another person's health. That's pretty heavy if you are a parent or have a partner who is unhealthy. You really must learn to love and care for yourself. Your family is counting on you to show they how to take care of themselves. You are their role model.

If your significant other is a priority over your own wellbeing, your body will oblige you. And no doubt has for years. It will continue to bow to your will in this until you are sick and or dead.

Please understand when I talk about someone having your best interests at heart, I am speaking of your long term best interests. It is easy to "give into someone" and get the KFC chicken for them when they are crying. At the time, that might seem like it makes the situation better. But in the long run, it perpetuates the problem. Look long term for yourself. Look long term for those you love. Shortsightedness is a huge problem in our culture. And because weight gain isn't instantaneous, and obesity related diseases do not happen overnight, we sometimes overlook them for the short term rewards.

It is easy to drink too much coffee when in the short term we are rewarded with being alert during a boring meeting. It is a lot more difficult to be self disciplined enough to turn off the TV and go to sleep at an hour that will ensure you a restful day tomorrow. More insidious than that is the brain chemistry that takes place when we drink diet colas. The brain rush is intoxicating for a short time, then in the aftermath it kills brain cells. I think of it like brain cell fireworks that burst into beautiful colors for a few seconds and then burn out when their colors fade. In the short term you don't notice the dead brain cells, but in the long run you may see problems with memory, cognitive function, etc. In the long term you will care, even if you don't now.

Intimacy is impossible without authenticity. If you are willing to be isolated in the short term to protect your long term mental and physical health, your priorities will repay you in spades in the coming years. I know a woman about 40 years old who does not make herself a priority, despite the fact that she works in the fitness industry. She fears isolation and her life choices prove it. She has five children and she is rarely if ever without a partner in her life. She is driven never to be alone, even for a short amount of time. The problem with that is that she settles for partners who hurt her both physically and emotionally, simply to avoid being alone.

Long term isolation is not healthy. But that does not mean that in order to be healthy you must be intimate with someone at all times. Balance and long term thinking are key here.

Periods of isolation can have some perks. These times allows you to be self reflective and to work on your own priorities without having to consider someone else. It allows you to get to know yourself as an independent individual. So many of us who are married have become the sum of our union. Our speech reflects it. It is "we" and "us" and many people have stopped thinking of us as individuals. In fact, I think we don't think of ourselves as separate individuals especially as we age together. We are so intertwined in our relationships that we only envision ourselves that way. It's a good thing when the relationship is healthy to be intimate. But intimacy does not mean losing who you are to another. And one day you will lose that partner. Then if you do not know who you are as an individual you may have a long struggle ahead of you.

I had my wedding tattoo design (yes instead of a ring I have a tattoo) based on the concept of the joining of two whole individuals. It is a Celtic Knot design with one heart in the center. If you look closely at the heart, you will see that it contains two whole and completely separate parts that together make up the one heart. That, in my humble opinion is the ultimate symbol for a healthy relationship.

Why is intimacy so important? It is important first because without deep personal human connections, thriving is unsustainable. Notice, I did not say "life is unsustainable". You can literally live without others, assuming you buy everything from the internet and never leave your home. It has been done. But that is not thriving. It is not ideal. It is not a real, authentic life. We are social beings, even the most introverted of us. Psychologically we need one another to thrive as much or more than we need the cycles of night and day.

If you have yet to make your life partnership choices, choose someone whose concern and care for you extends to the long term. Choose someone who cares about their own health and wellbeing and by extension yours. Pick a partner who has your long term best interests at heart.

If you have already made your life partnership choices, use your behavior to model good health to your family. Work as a team toward a healthy life. If you are in an unsafe relationship, talk to someone who can help you. Psychologists are great for this! If you are being abused, find a way out. If you need help but don't know what to do to safely get out, most states have something called 'One Call' that can literally save your life. It is free, and they can help in a variety of ways. Call someone for help before it is too late.

If your partner is unhealthy by choice, you may need to stop enabling them. By not enabling your partner to continue to be unhealthy, you are showing them that you love them. Make healthy meals for yourself, and your family (I'm not just talking to women here- this goes for everyone). They might complain about it at first, but remember that everything is an acquired taste. Eventually they will come around. Do what is right for you, it will be right for them in the long run. Work toward a healthy intimacy with your partner, if at all possible.

If you do not create a healthy intimate relationship with someone, you risk long term isolation. Keep in mind, an unhealthy relationship is just as isolating as no intimacy at all.

By the same token, if you do not create a healthy intimacy with food, you risk the isolation of obesity and the diseases that often accompany it. This is where the rubber meets the road. Is your relationship to food a healthy one? Or is it a sick one? Are you hiding food? Do you eat alone so that no one knows exactly how much you have eaten? Do you use food for comfort? Do you use food for any reason other than nutrition? Does food fuel your health or your destruction? Only you can answer these questions.

We've really got to give food a break. It was never meant as a tool to help us with our psychological pain, restlessness, or boredom. It is and forever will be fuel. That is all. It has no power to comfort you. Advertising companies have anthropomorphized food to the point where Dough Boys and raisins sing and dance around our TV screens. They exude the warmth of a hug, and bake us "happy" according to ad execs. Coffee is "the best part of waking up" and sharing Twizzlers is an intimate act shared between lovers. Speaking of love, chocolate is at the top of the "food is love" pyramid.

Sharing Life

In our culture we no longer know how to share our lives and celebrate without food. What would a celebration without food look like? I challenge you to plan a celebration where there is no food or caloric drinks (maybe just water). What about an activity outdoors together to celebrate something? Maybe when your kid graduates from third grade (or college) you could do an outdoor challenge together as a group of family and friends that would be symbolic of their accomplishments. Make up creative invitations that call for everyone to undertake an afternoon adventure that celebrates the kind of work it takes to achieve a goal like college (or third grade) graduation. Take a 5 mile hike as a group! If Grandma can't go that far, give her the job of sitting at a water station half way through and supporting the team or driving the broom wagon.

And if you love to sit around with your friends on a Saturday night watching silly old movies playing drinking games, what about instead of taking in all those empty calories you could do something completely different and have a blast? What about every time you see the gopher (especially if he's dancing) during Caddyshack, you do a 30 second dance party? Any mention of the gopher by any name including names other than gopher (varmint, for example) you change places with your friends. Every time a golf club is swung... get up and swing an imaginary club! You set the rules. Just have fun without the extra calories! Double plus: no next morning hangover! You might be a little sore from the exercise if you are new to movement, but it is worth it! Serve ants on a log (celery with hazelnut butter as an homage to the floating candy bar), fizzy water with coconut shavings and a lemon twist with little umbrellas and require summer golf attire!

My point is that we not only make the changes that we know are fundamental, but that we re-examine the traditions we hold dear. We celebrate 11 Federal holidays a year in America. Those do not include an annual Superbowl party, Birthdays, Anniversaries, Valentine's Day, Cinco de Mayo, St. Patrick's Day, Mardi Gras, Mother or Father's Day, Halloween, Christmas Eve, New Year's Eve, Memorial Day, Labor Day, graduations, other personal accomplishments, or any additional religious holidays that involve food. Add those up and we are celebrating something involving food 3 times a month, many of us more than that! The average extra calories taken in at a birthday party, for example, is 500 calories. Eggnog at each of the Christmas parties you attend is about 360 calories per cup. If you "let go" on Thanksgiving or the Superbowl you can add 4000 calories at each of those celebrations! Add up the results of food based celebrations throughout the year and you wind up with 54,000 calories at 3 celebrations per month. (I took the average calories for a Thanksgiving (highest) and a birthday party (lowest) and averaged them together. Then added up three a month. That's an extra 15 pounds a year!! For many of us, that's a pretty conservative estimate. That's nothing to celebrate!

Part of the reason we have talked about the various online programs is so that you can develop a program for yourself based on evidence. This is the evidence that what you are doing is promoting and reinforcing your health. There is no substitute for having an individualized program, based on the evidence of what works for you.

Does your current diet increase your weight, or allow for the maintenance of a weight that is healthy for you? Is that good or bad for you? This is not a one size fits all program. Despite what they say, no program is. Unless your program is tailored to you personally, you are using a one size fits all solution. We all know those only work for 2% of the population. They should really call them 'one size fits 2%' to be realistic.

I have a hunch that you know some of the things that work for you. I know, for example, that eating fish agrees with me and that the fewer grains I eat the better I feel. Gluten especially bothers me, but until I was able to study my own dietary habits I could not tell how what I ate was affecting me.

Write Your Story

Make a note of all the things that you have done that contributed to your health and to a healthy weight.

Get to know someone you respect better. Spend more time with a person you want to be more like. What is it that you respect about them?

Make notes about your personal changes over a few week's time.

Talk to the significant people in your life about your transition to health and wholeness. Afterward, write down the results of those chats.

What is the state of your intimate relationships?

Describe your most intimate relationship including its problems and successes.

What could be improved as it relates to health and longevity?

Challenge yourself to find alternatives to unhealthy celebrations and ongoing activities and practices. What is coming up (a wedding, birthday, etc.) that you could change to help you incorporate your new healthy identity?

Are your past intimate relationships still hurting you?

What are you doing to confront those issues?

How do you comfort yourself when they rear their ugly heads?

The next time a hurt comes up, keep track of what you use for comfort. Is it the healthiest way to comfort yourself?

What do intimacy and comfort have to do with one another?

While intimacy can be a comfort, intimacy abused can send you in search of comfort for a lifetime.

Design a comfort activity and practice it. Use that instead of food or drink when you need comfort.

Keep a log of your motivations for choosing the foods you eat over the next 2 weeks. For example, this morning I had broccoli and onions and mushrooms for purely nutritional purposes. I wish I was so clear headed about every single choice I make. For example, last evening I ate an entire dark chocolate bar for a treat because it was the anniversary of a day on which I had been severely mistreated.

Using any number of different tools available you can log these motivations, see patterns and get to the bottom of your most likely food triggers.

Further, take some time after your choice to write a bit about what it meant for you. My dark chocolate bar was a psychological way for me to even the score between mistreatment and positive experiences. Yet, food, no matter how good for you, can never even the score.

STAGE SEVEN: CARE

I have mentioned that I taught a 'learn to run' class through an athletic shoe store and the great sense of connection and fulfillment that gave me. The focus of this stage is not directly on you. The focus is on your care for others. When you have gone through all the preceding stages and you have lost your weight and begun to maintain it you may feel like your job is finished. However, the thing that is most telling about us is how we show our care for others.

What we give to the next generation is a vital part of our own narrative.

This is the place where a lot of people fail and regain their weight. Self focus is good, but it must be followed up with a genuine concern for giving back to complete the circle of our lives. Without this the other stages may simply collapse in on us.

When you give to others of your own experience and knowledge it is a powerful experience not only for them but also for you. Not only does it keep you focused on some aspect of healthy behavior (leading a walking group, for example) but it reinforces in you that what you have done is now a part of your identity. This for me is the most beautiful stage. And you do not have to wait until you have overcome obesity to do it. Acting in a type of faith (if you will) you can reach out to others and give no matter where you are.

Make giving your practice. Give something of your new identity to others. I'm not telling you that in order to keep your weight off everyone must become a personal trainer. If that is your passion, go for it! Find something of your experience that has held meaning for you and use that to give. Give from an authentic place that gives you joy. If you find that you really enjoy healthy cooking, teach a cooking class to seniors (either the high school or aging variety!) through your community education extension. There are always opportunities to teach in community ed.

Maybe your passion is simply something you love to do that you now have more energy to pursue! Share that with others! Find a way to be civically minded, form a group to help clean up trash in an area of town that needs it. Everyone has something they can share with their community. Take time...make time to do it.

It is vital to your own development that you give.

All this giving will leave you with a sense of accomplishment and productivity. You will gain self respect and maybe the respect of others too! But what happens when you fail to give of your experience to others is that you will be left with a dissatisfaction with the process in general. You will not experience the richness of success, instead you will feel stagnate.

In caring for others you may need to take a bit to time for some self care here too. Every person who has lived has made mistakes and maybe some decisions they regret. Take some time to allow yourself that reality. Allow for the mistakes as a part of the human learning experience. We learn good judgement from bad judgment they say. If I had to do this life over again there are a few things I would definitely do differently. When I think about all I have put my body through over the years by not dealing with this disease, it makes me sad. I have squandered and abused this precious gift called health. However I know that it is vitally important that I also forgive myself for all that. We can't go back in time (until the "way back machine" is a reality) so going forward I will afford myself grace. Grace to know that life does not happen in a vacuum. Grace to know that in surviving the trials and tribulations of life I did what I needed to do in order to emotionally survive. I make a pledge, as I hope you will too, to care for myself from here until I can once again experience vitality.

I asked the question in chapter 21, 'what's new?' This stage is the demonstration of that question fulfilled. It is a way to continue to keep renewing your commitment to a healthy life. Maybe what you give is indirect. Not everyone is a natural born teacher. And not everyone wants to get up in front of a crowd. And you don't have to! Find what comes naturally and do that. Maybe you are a great listener and as a result you start a support group for people who want to share their stories and encourage one another. Maybe you write a book! Maybe you paint, or just clean for people who can no longer do it for themselves. Maybe you pick one other person each year who you encourage and mentor toward a healthier, more authentic life.

Get involved and stay involved. There is no better payoff in the world than when you give of yourself to someone else.

Write Your Story

What are the needs in your community, as they relate to health and wellness? I am not necessarily referring to your town. I am talking about the people in your world, those around you.

Is there something you can do that would contribute to the health and wellness of others?

Do you have an assisted living home in your neighborhood or city? They can always use enthusiastic volunteers. Maybe organize a sitting exercise class, or a walk for the residents. Find out what they need by talking to the administration there.

Who are you mentoring this year? If you are like me and can't get out a lot, you could mentor someone online.

If you have a teenager you could work together on a project for community wellness. Find a way to work together in a helping capacity. Nothing bridges gaps like meeting the needs of others.

Write a short pledge to yourself to care, protect, and honor yourself. Stick it on the fridge, or on a note in your cubical. Be proud of who you are becoming, and of who you have been.

Now write a pledge to care for someone outside your normal circle of friends and family. It doesn't have to be big, just some way to reach out beyond yourself.

STAGE EIGHT: INTEGRITY

This is the final stage in the development of who you are becoming. It may not happen for many years, but it is important to be mindful of it as it speaks to your choices throughout all the other stages and throughout your life. In your life as you navigate the various stages of development that result in your authentic healthy life, you will enter a point at which you become self reflective. You will have a chance to contemplate your choices and your experiences from the perspective of someone who is winding down and bringing closure to that experience.

Like I said, this will probably happen many years down the road. Do not get the mistaken idea that these stages are something you do as a quick fix for obesity. They are not. Nowhere near. But some stages will be quite quick, while others take years. The idea is that you continue to develop throughout your life. You continue to write your narrative until you die. How much better is it to be deliberate about it? You can be who you want to be, and it can be reflected in your experiences, the way you interact with others, and the way you guide the next generation.

It is a happy thought to get to the end of your life to be able to look back on it with pride and confidence that you lived a vibrant full life. This is where you gain integrity. A lot of folks think that integrity is doing something with honor. That is one definition. But this is a more holistic way of looking at integrity. Having made deliberately positive decisions you are able to look at your life as having integrity. Authenticity and integrity go hand in hand and both manifest in this stage. It may not mean much to you if you are in the first stages of your new narrative. But as you progress through those stages you must understand that this final stage is coming, whether or not you are aware of it. Better to be aware of it and live deliberately in preparation for it than to live in ignorance of it.

From time to time I say to people that my goal in life is to have the best stories in the nursing home. True. That is my overarching life goal. I live my life in as deliberate a manner as is possible, so that I have developed my narrative to its fullest. I want to live life on my terms, with the ability to look back on my experiences with a smile.

Contentment is highly underrated. That is the reward of this stage. It is the culmination of all the other stages and their rewards. When you have found your path, and you know you can completely trust it, you can begin moving through the stages. Since that is stage one, it is your first task. Study what diet and exercise routines work for you and when you find it, make it a practice in your life. Be as devoted to it as if it were your own child because it will save your life. My son uses a phrase I like a lot: Be a 365 day monk. The image is that of someone focused and devoted completely and without reservation. You can only do this if you know from the evidence that your program is right for you.

In the next stage you change everything you have been doing that is unhealthy and replace it with what is right for you. Shed the illusion that you above being typical and build your own process that actually works for you. You can be certain because your program was designed around you, not some health guru or expert who is trying to sell you protein powder or raspberry keytones. You are unique and your story is important. You must position yourself to tell the story of your life that you want to tell. You must position yourself to live the life you want to live, without regret or reservation. Take responsibility for who you are and who you are becoming. Be deliberate.

You will know you have begun to develop who you want to be by the amount of 'push back' you get from others. This is a good sign. Social changes do not happen without some amount of push back. Neither do individual changes. When you see those around you becoming a little uncomfortable, take heart. Change is difficult, not just for you but for those around you.

Entering into maturity means that you must decide if you are a producer or a consumer in this life. If you are a consumer, your focus in life is on taking and using. If you are a producer your focus is on giving and creating. This is the definition of growing up. You must shed your childlike mannerisms and move toward your adult life. Becoming a producer is significant in terms of keeping your weight under control because you cannot be both a producer and a consumer. You will focus on one or the other. Being a consumer will literally keep you tied to the disease of obesity, while being a producer will make it possible for you shed the diagnosis and become who you really want to be. You can be a shortsighted child, or a mature individual who cares about the future.

Your identity is all you really have when it comes down to it. In the final assessment of your life you will leave behind an imprint. This imprint is your narrative. Living a life that can be reflected in the eyes of others is what being authentic is all about. When your body, mind, and personal narrative all come together in harmony you have created your new identity. Being vibrant and fully alive is what life is all about. We cannot be vibrant when our bodies are weighed down by not just the physical insecurities and weaknesses, but the mental ones that walk hand in hand with an obese body. As you begin to truly shed the excess "childhood fat" and childish thinking and you begin to gain muscle you will also gain a sense of personal strength and security that comes with it. It is this strength that will enable you to fight for what you know you want for yourself against all odds and against Temptation.

You can only defend what you know you have. If you are secure in your progress and you have shed the childish ways that originally married you to obesity, you can then face the world with confidence. You can only integrate with the rest of the world if you are strong enough and if you truly know who you are and where you are going. Without this stage, trying to integrate your new identity with the rest of the world will cause you will flail. The biggest reason to be aware of the final stage in this developmental sequence is to know where you are going! Without that, you will flail, Temptation will have her way with you and you will remain a child for the rest of your days. Which by extension means that you will also remain connected to obesity no matter how hard you struggle or white knuckle it.

You cannot give what you do not possess. If you have and you do not give, you live in emotional poverty. Much of life is a paradox. That is the nature of giving. It is when we give of ourselves that our rewards are the richest. Writing a check isn't the same thing. It may be valuable, no question. But giving of ourselves gives us a sense of satisfaction and contentment that is something far beyond material rewards. It is the fulfillment of our contract with the universe. It is our solemn duty to give what we have learned to the future.

Integrity is the result of a life well lived. That is the goal. If obesity and ill health do not stop you from experiencing life to its fullest, you have nothing to worry about. For me, the ideal is to be whole and healthy, integrating my thoughts and values into my life in a vibrant, authentic expression I can share with others.

Write Your Story

Spend just a bit of time and imagine what people might say at your funeral. Write out a short speech that the person closest to you in life could read about you.

Write out a short dialogue between two of your past co-workers, friends, or relatives that might happen at your funeral.

Now re-write those same speeches with your goals in mind. What would like people to say about you that they cannot yet say about your life?

How does that change your perspective on your life's choices?

THE 'YOU-SHAPED' DIET

The biggest complaint that I have heard about diet books and programs is a lack of real content. It is important to me that you have all the tools you will need in order to be successful. If you are to stop mimicking the diet and exercise gurus you must have a concrete way to study your own behavior and to create your own program. The heart of this program is to create a perfectly suited, evidence based program that works for you, for life. The only way to do that is to study your own behaviors and see what works. It is that simple. But since most of us are not research scientists (and have no desire to be) we must be able to do this in practical real world terms. In a perverse way I am inspired by the government's attempts at a nutrition chart. A number of years back the government put out a new food pyramid what was so confusing almost no one understood it. Since then I think that despite the great efforts of Michelle Obama, Americans are still confused about what is good for us. I do think that the most confusing food pyramid was aiming at something important. It was trying to say that since we are all different, with differing nutritional needs, we each need a customized program. Don't get me wrong, I don't think they successfully said that. But I think it was their aim. My point is that there is NO ONE SIZE FITS ALL SOLUTION. We must all take responsibility, understand our own health position, and work within our own reality to better our health. There is no one thing called a "diet" that works magic when you eat it. There is no one way to eat to become healthier and leaner. There is what's right for you and what's right for me. And it is different for every person on the planet. So, grow up and put some real effort into it. Find out what you need and do what's right for you.

Baseline

First, understand that this is not brain surgery. This is simple, there are just a lot of moving parts. Using the questions at the end of each chapter you can start choosing what is most urgent for you to understand about yourself. First, take stock in your diet and exercise practices. Keep logs of what you do using the suggestions given in this text. This is foundational. Take a month (a whole month?! Yes, a whole month!) and keep track of everything you eat and every time you exercise. Along with that, log your emotional reactions to your life and how it relates to your food choices in a journal format. Log your daily resting pulse, weekly blood pressure, weekly weight, daily accounts of your own productivity, energy, mood, every measure of your health you can get your hands on. You can ask your doctor what blood tests they have run recently and include things like cholesterol levels, inflammation markers, blood sugars, complete blood counts, thyroid counts, measurements in inches, etc. These are generally run annually during your physical. In addition, take note on a daily basis at least, of any symptoms like being chronically tired, or thirsty, etc., and show your log to your doctor. This provides them with a wealth of information with which to help you toward improving your health.

I like to use a spreadsheet to keep my log. There are lots of ways to do this, just choose one that is comfortable for you. For a time I used http://www.patientslikeme.com/ to track my RA and thyroid symptoms. It was really helpful to both me and my docs.

That is what we will call baseline. Measure your baseline numbers against the health indicators your doctor uses. You can find them online, or through your doc. There is usually a range for each health indicator that is considered healthy. For example, you know your blood pressure but do you know what a healthy blood pressure for someone your age is? What kind of inflammation markers are normal for someone of your age and build? What effects inflammation markers? What will you do to lower yours?

Create a chart with your baseline markers and compare them to the healthy markers. In this way you will know for certain what your health goals are. Just knowing that you have obesity is no where near enough to understand you own health goals. Yet that is the only information that is important to the diet gurus!! You have all seen the ads! "How much do you want to lose?" They have made it the only goal, yet it is far from telling in terms of health. And trusting them to do what is right for you is dangerous!

Your baseline is important because it is a clear picture of where you are now. Understanding that you have the disease of obesity is stage zero. It tells you so little that it doesn't rise to the point of being a significant health goal in and of itself. Yes it is important, but it is by no means the whole story of your health.

You can't possibly know where you are going without knowing where you are right now. Think of it in terms of a trip. If you don't have a starting place, getting directions is impossible. Yet every single day people begin new diet and exercise programs without taking stock of where they are starting. They take directions without any idea where they are starting, how long it might take them to get there, or if the destination is actually a place they want to go! In reality, if your baseline shows you are a type two diabetic with high blood pressure, you would need to know that kind of thing in order to avoid certain kinds of diets that would be more harmful than good for you! What's worse is you are not really given enough information about what diets are good for different kinds of health goal. How can you hope to make an informed decision? For example, if you have high blood sugar a diet high in carbohydrates is not appropriate for you. But it sounds healthy on paper to be a vegetarian, for example. And the media is very convincing! But a vegetarian diet is (generally speaking) a high carbohydrate diet which could easily cause you more health issues than it solves! But the advocates for that diet are often busy telling you how damaging animal products are for your health, leaving out the part about the high carbohydrate issue that could contribute to diabetic complications if you are not careful. But for someone with high cholesterol, a vegetarian diet could be life saving! It pays to know your own baseline! Diet gurus are going to assume that you fit the model for their diet and that it is appropriate for everyone. They Are Wrong. It is up to you to know if it is wrong for you because the guru won't tell you. Remember they want your money. They aren't going to tell you that their diet is potentially harmful if it means losing them money!

Dare to Compare!

Once you have a good handle on your baseline you can see the condition of your health. It is like a snap shot in time of how you are doing. When we have a baseline of one month's work we can compare it to what health looks like on paper. We know the range of numbers that represent health, so when you see that your cholesterol is 230 you can see right away that something might be wrong and that you must dig further in order to know what each number is, good versus bad cholesterol, triglycerides, the size and stickiness of the cells, etc. These tests are commonly available and your medical doctor, or a naturopathic doctor should be able to order them for you if you need more info. No matter what test results you are looking at, if you have a number that is above the healthy range, dig in! Do some research about the kinds of things you need to know about high blood sugar or triglycerides or cholesterol, etc. This is your life!! Know your numbers! Know what they mean in comparison to healthy numbers!! Take a note book (or a voice recorder) to the doctor's office, take notes and ask for copies of lab results each time. The healthy levels are usually right there in the lab test reports! Don't forget to share your logs and concerns with your doctor. I have made copies for my docs to put into their files. I don't sleep well because of the pain I encounter at night. When that started I opened a new log with all kinds of info about my sleep habits, medications, what kinds of supplements I was taking, and the routines I tried to get to sleep and stay asleep, etc. When you have a concern, create a "study" of that part of your life. Sleep hygiene is an evolving and powerful field that is really helpful for people like me who find it hard to get enough sleep. Information is power, and by studying my own sleep patterns, nighttime routines, etc. I was able to tap into a vast amount of information about sleep hygiene. I still don't always get enough sleep, but I have a lot more in the way of tools to help me with the problem.

Create a Plan

Now that you know your numbers and how they stack up, take some time to talk to your doctor about what approach you should take. Ask about the kinds of foods that you should be avoiding. Don't just jump to heavy duty meds before you explore what dietary changes might be able to do for you. There are dire situations which require meds for these problems, but in general you should be adjusting your lifestyle to address those problems anyway! Talk to your doctor, and if you feel you can't talk to them, change doctors! If you, like me, struggle with high triglycerides, you might not know a lot about that. I had never heard that term when I was first told it was a problem for me. Triglycerides are part of your overall cholesterol number. Many people who have obesity struggle with this symptomless yet potentially dangerous heart related problem. If you do, there are things you can do to help lower triglycerides. Limiting your fat and sugars is important. Not eating more calories than you burn daily is another important consideration. Keep in mind that I am highlighting some of the most common problems that people who suffer with obesity face. This is not an exhaustive list by any means. Talk with your doctor about your health indicators to be sure you are covering your bases.

The great thing about keeping these kinds of records is that you can easily see your progress. As your blood levels, blood pressure, resting pulse, etc. begin to come down you can see it right away! That's motivating to me! And if you are making changes and you do not see evidence of these problems resolving, you can be sure that you may have to re-evaluate your strategy.

Also talk with your doc about how long it might take to correct the problems you have, like lowering your cholesterol, or your blood sugar, etc. You should have a realistic notion about how long it takes to effect these issues so you don't lose heart in the process.

Keep in mind, many health indicators do not change over night. You will have to be patient and tenacious in your attempts to improve your health and vitality. But the rewards are great when you improve these markers just a little! Losing just 10% of your excess body fat can help drop blood pressure, blood sugars, and a whole host of other health markers. Every little bit helps. And you can see now how easy it is! It is just a matter of subtraction! If your cholesterol is 230, for example, you are going to find that the medical community suggests that a healthy level is under 200. What will you do to encourage those numbers to go down? Find out what kinds of foods you eat that contain cholesterol (all animal foods) and severely limit those. You will want to eat foods that you know encourage the numbers to decrease like whole grain oats for example. Some strategies will include increased exercise and movement of all kinds. For example, to lower your resting pulse you will want to increase aerobic exercise. I love this health marker because it says a lot about your fitness levels. Similarly your recovery rate after exercise is very telling. How long does it take to go from an elevated heart rate during exercise to a recovered heart rate? The longer it takes, the less fit you are. Maybe your strategy includes shortening your heart rate recovery times.

Your plan should include as many different strategies as necessary to lower the most emergent problem areas in your health profile. If you have high blood pressure, a high resting heart rate, high triglycerides, and obesity create a strategy that encompasses all these problems. Choose a diet that is appropriate to help lower your triglycerides and an exercise plan that will lower your resting pulse and blood pressure.

How do you know what diet or fitness program to choose? Follow the evidence, not the latest fad. Simply look at your baseline markers and your symptoms and make sure that you understand which of the indicators are troublesome. For example, high blood sugars indicate that you may need to lower your intake of carbohydrates, especially simple sugars. You can use reliable online tools like http://www.webmd.com or http://www.mayoclinic.org to search for info about your trouble spots or talk to your doctor about options. If you use the web, be careful to choose reliable sources that are based in science and not wishful thinking, fads, or selling you a product. Money is the biggest indicator that a website is unreliable. If you ask yourself "what are they selling?" and the answer is easy to see, hop off that website and look somewhere else. And stay away from ads. They are ALL ABOUT THE MONEY not about your health. You might be tempted to click on the "lose belly fat" ads if this is a problem area for you. Don't do it! It's just an ad, not science! While we are talking about the media in general, do not trust newspaper statistics. That's right. Do not trust them. I read online new stories about health studies all the time and every single time I do I get really angry because journalists are not generally trained in the interpretation of statistics. Most of what they say makes no sense at all! For example, the will say something like "Five out of six patients were better after their heart stent surgery". Better than WHAT? Well, they don't say! That's just one example of what goes out via the media every day! Put it all out of your mind. If you want to know what the research says, google the actual research study and read it for yourself. If you have questions about it, email the authors! They are real people who are generally gracious enough to answer your earnest questions about their work. The media is famous for getting this kind of thing wrong. My first stats class in grad school had us looking at all the major new sources and analyzing their stories that contained statistics. It was a constant giggle-a-thon because 99% of it made no sense at all! It's not that they are "twisting the stats" to make them say something specific. The papers are just clueless! So, until they have earned our trust, get your health information straight from the researchers themselves. And get it from your doctor and from your own study of your health. Trends and fads are dangerous. This is one area you don't want to be on the cutting edge of!

If your numbers are all good and you have no symptoms you are in luck (and probably quite young). But if you have obesity, you know that at least one number is not healthy: your weight. In that case you know that you can simply lower the amount of calories you eat and increase the number of calories you burn. It is simple, but for folks who have no co-morbidities and no unhealthy test results or problematic symptoms, all indications are that you are doing something right. Keep it up, and just modify your calories on both ends.

Let's talk about the psychological processes in the book. Keeping a journal is going to be important. As you read through this book you will notice that many of the chapters include questions or prompts that are designed to help you journal your psychological experiences as you lose the weight and improve your health. If you are using ibooks you can simply keep notes within the pages of the book. I prefer to keep an electronic journal on my laptop or a physical blank book. Whatever your preference it is therapeutic to keep notes and write down your stories from each of the psychological stages. This will help you to visualize your progression through the stages, which will reinforce your growth and maturity toward your new identity.

The medical problems associated with obesity generally show up in groups. The wonderful thing is that for those of us with obesity, solutions to individual problems will likely have a positive effect on the entire group of related problems. If you are doing your bit to lower your cholesterol, you will likely also effect your weight and possibly your blood sugar too. Triglycerides and blood sugars are related, as are blood pressure, resting pulse, and cholesterol. Your mental health and psychological development is related to all these problems. Improve one and get a multiplied effect! That's powerful good news!

But be honest. It does you no good to live in denial. You are really only hurting yourself. For example, you may be eating a "clean" diet but way too much of it. You may think that your vegan diet is ideal because you love animals and want to save the environment. But if you are eating a vegan diet and gaining weight, something is wrong. Those are the kinds of indicators you should be looking for. Many people gain weight on perfectly healthy diets that are inappropriate for them. Someone who needs fewer carbs and more protein may not do well on a vegan diet, no matter their philosophy. That doesn't mean that you need to eat meat. It might mean that you need to stop eating processed foods like breads, cookies and chips. This is at the heart of the problem in a society that follows diet gurus based on how they look. Following someone else's diet is simply childish pretending. At best it is mimicry. Just because it worked for them, doesn't mean it will work for you. Just because they are ripped and lean does not mean you will be. And just because they are persuasive does not mean that they know what they are talking about or that they know what is good for you. They do not know you or your health history, your body's needs, allergies, psychological health, co-morbidities or anything else about you. But you can know all that and you can build the perfect evidence-based program for your health.

Hippocrates, the father of modern medicine said, "Let food be thy medicine and medicine be thy food"

Food can be your medicine. It can go a long way toward healing you, in some cases it is far more effective than drugs. Use it the way you would medicine, be diligent and mindful about what you eat and how it will effect your body and your maladies. It is difficult to see a sugary pastry as medicine, isn't it? If you have high cholesterol you must find out by researching your own blood samples if when you eat meat it increases your cholesterol. Test it for 3 or 6 months. Take a blood sample, eat meat for 3 or 6 months and test your blood again. Then if you want to eat a big steak you know first hand whether or not you will pay a price in terms of damage to your body. If you have seen that happen in your own records, you can be sure of what will happen when you eat that steak. For five years I ate at steady diet of zucchini, cheese and turkey ham in a little hot dish. After one year of that, my cholesterol was 127 and stayed that way for as long as I ate that meal consistently. I also ran 5 miles a day. Know your own body and how it reacts to different foods and movement. It really is that simple. Think long term, like an adult.

Once you have the evidence of your health snapshot, done your due diligence to find out what kind of nutrition program would best address your health needs, you need to think about your physical limitations. You need to create as part of your plan a way to move. If you have co-morbidities be sure to consider them in your plans. I have RA and fibromyalgia so I can no longer run. It's simple. But it is more important to know what I can do. What kind of movement is best for you if you have diseases or conditions in addition to obesity? To accommodate my co-morbidities I swim and when I can I walk. I use exercises that don't further destroy my joints or cause me more pain. Create a movement plan that makes you feel good. Do it as consistently as you eat. Daily. Consider it part of your health plan to combat the disease of obesity.

You've seen your numbers and created your goals, now it is just a matter of follow through. Work at it. Manage your disease, because obesity is a disease that demands management. It is not enough to pay attention to it for a month and then slip back into old habits. You know that you have a disease that will kill you if you continue to act that way. So Grow up. Eat your veggies. Move your butt. Be who you want to be, today. Don't wait for someone to rescue you because there may not be time for a rescue. I have heard it said that often the first symptom of heart disease is death. If you know your body, your blood counts, etc. you will (more than likely) not have to worry about being surprised by a heart attack. You are your best and in truth your only advocate. Be the rescue you need.

Managing the disease is about regularly monitoring your program to be sure it is working. As you age you will need to tweak your program to accommodate your body's changes. Simply add monitoring to your schedule, as you would if you were a diabetic monitoring your blood sugar. I keep it in my calendar in order to remind myself that I have to check my numbers. If your program is working you will see results. Forge ahead! If not you will see confusing numbers and a lack of progress. At that point it is time for a change. Go back and compile a new baseline. Be sure you know where you are and compare it to where you have been and to what is healthy. From there the picture will become clear and you will know what to change.

I honestly hope you will share your stories with me! I'd love to hear from you about your progress and what works for you and why! Email me at carrieon@mac.com or go online to my website http://www.fromheretovitality.com/.

GLOSSARY

ANECDOTAL
A limited selection of examples which support or refute an argument, but which are not supported by scientific or statistical analysis.

Anecdotal evidence is an informal account of evidence in the form of an anecdote. The term is often used in contrast to scientific evidence, as evidence that cannot be investigated using the scientific method. The problem with arguing based on anecdotal evidence is that anecdotal evidence is not necessarily typical; only statistical evidence can determine how typical something is. Misuse of anecdotal evidence is a logical fallacy.

For more about anecdotes and anecdotal evidence:
http://en.wikipedia.org/wiki/Anecdotes

ASSIMILATION
To absorb and incorporate one thing into another.
For Example:
▪ Photosynthesis, a process whereby carbon dioxide and water are transformed into a number of organic molecules in plant cells.
▪ Nitrogen fixation from the soil into organic molecules by symbiotic bacteria which live in the roots of certain plants, such as Leguminosae.
▪ Magnesium supplements orotate, oxide, sulfate, citrate, and glycerate are all structurally similar. However, oxide and sulfate are not water soluble and do not enter the blood stream while orotate and glycerate have normal exiguous liver conversion. Chlorophyll sources or magnesium citrate are highly bioassimilable.
▪ The absorption of nutrients into the body after digestion in the intestine and its transformation in biological tissues and fluids.
▪ Assimilation is occurring in every cell of the body to help develop new cells.
http://en.wikipedia.org/wiki/Assimilation_%28biology%29

BINGE
Indulge in an activity, esp. eating, to excess
some dieters say they cannot help binging on chocolate.
Compulsive overeating, (COE) characteristic of binge eating disorder, in which people tend to eat more than necessary resulting in more stress. This is mainly caused by 'binge eating disorder.

(Google Dictionary, 2012,
http://en.wikipedia.org/wiki/Eating_disorder)

BIOAVAILABLE
The ease with which something is absorbed from the digestive tract. The higher the bioavailability, the greater the total absorption and rate of absorption.
(http://www.naturallyfit-supplements.com/terms-you-need-to-know/)
In pharmacology, bioavailability is used to describe the fraction of an administered dose of unchanged drug that reaches the systemic circulation, one of the principal pharmacokinetic properties of drugs. ...
(http://en.wikipedia.org/wiki/Bioavailable)

BLOOD PRESSURE
Sometimes referred to as arterial blood pressure, is the pressure exerted by circulating blood upon the walls of blood vessels, and is one of the principal vital signs. When used without further specification, "blood pressure" usually refers to the arterial pressure of the systemic circulation. During each heartbeat, blood pressure varies between a maximum (systolic) and a minimum (diastolic) pressure.[1] The blood pressure in the circulation is principally due to the pumping action of the heart.[2] Differences in mean blood pressure are responsible for blood flow from one location to another in the circulation. The rate of mean blood flow depends on the resistance to flow presented by the blood vessels. Mean blood pressure decreases as the circulating blood moves away from the heart through arteries and capillaries due to viscous losses of energy. Mean blood pressure drops over the whole circulation, although most of the fall occurs along the small arteries and arterioles.[3] Gravity affects blood pressure via hydrostatic forces (e.g., during standing) and valves in veins, breathing, and pumping from contraction of skeletal muscles also influence blood pressure in veins.[2]
The measurement blood pressure without further specification usually refers to the systemic arterial pressure measured at a person's upper arm and is a measure of the pressure in the brachial artery, major artery in the upper arm. A person's blood pressure is usually expressed in terms of the systolic pressure over diastolic pressure and is measured in millimetres of mercury (mmHg), for example 120/80.

http://en.wikipedia.org/wiki/Blood_pressure

BLOOD SUGAR

The blood sugar concentration or blood glucose level is the amount of glucose (sugar) present in the blood of a human or animal. The body naturally tightly regulates blood glucose levels as a part of metabolic homeostasis.

Glucose is the primary source of energy for the body's cells, and blood lipids (in the form of fats and oils) are primarily a compact energy store. (There are exceptions. For example, because their dietary metabolizable carbohydrates tend to be used by rumen organisms,[2] ruminants tend to be continuously gluconeogenic;[3] consequently their hepatocytes must rely on such primary energy sources as volatile fatty acids, absorbed from the rumen, rather than glucose.) Glucose is transported from the intestines or liver to body cells via the bloodstream, and is made available for cell absorption via the hormone insulin, produced by the body primarily in the pancreas.

The mean normal blood glucose level in humans is about 5.5 mM (5.5 mmol/L or 100 mg/dL, i.e. milligrams/deciliter);[4] however, this level fluctuates throughout the day. Glucose levels are usually lowest in the morning, before the first meal of the day (termed "the fasting level"), and rise after meals for an hour or two by a few millimolar. The normal blood glucose level (tested while fasting) for non-diabetics, should be between 70 and 100 milligrams per deciliter (mg/dL). Blood sugar levels for those without diabetes and who are not fasting should be below 125 mg/dL. [5] The blood glucose target range for diabetics, according to the American Diabetes Association, should be 70 - 130 (mg/dL) before meals, and less than 180 mg/dL after meals (as measured by a blood glucose monitor).[6]

Blood sugar levels outside the normal range may be an indicator of a medical condition. A persistently high level is referred to as hyperglycemia; low levels are referred to as hypoglycemia. Diabetes mellitus is characterized by persistent hyperglycemia from any of several causes, and is the most prominent disease related to failure of blood sugar regulation. A temporarily elevated blood sugar level may also result from severe stress, such as trauma, stroke, myocardial infarction, surgery, or illness[citation needed]. Intake of alcohol causes an initial surge in blood sugar, and later tends to cause levels to fall. Also, certain drugs can increase or decrease glucose levels.[7]
http://en.wikipedia.org/wiki/Blood_sugar

BMI
Body Mass Index: The result of dividing weight (in kilograms)
by height (in meters) squared [weight (kg)/height (m)2] (Okoro,
Sintler, & Khan, 2009).

BROOM WAGON
According to Wikipedia.com, "The Broom Wagon (not to be
confused with a Sag Wagon) is the name for the vehicle that follows
a Cycle Road Race picking up stragglers (or sweeping them up)
who are unable to make it to the finish of the race within the time
permitted."
I am applying the same concept to a long walk.

CHOLESTEROL LEVELS
According to the lipid hypothesis, abnormal cholesterol levels
(hypercholesterolemia) — that is, higher concentrations of LDL and
lower concentrations of functional HDL — are strongly associated
with cardiovascular disease because these promote atheroma
development in arteries (atherosclerosis). This disease process leads
to myocardial infarction (heart attack), stroke, and peripheral
vascular disease. Since higher blood LDL, especially higher LDL
particle concentrations and smaller LDL particle size, contribute to
this process more than the cholesterol content of the HDL
particles,[46] LDL particles are often termed "bad cholesterol"
because they have been linked to atheroma formation. On the other
hand, high concentrations of functional HDL, which can remove
cholesterol from cells and atheroma, offer protection and are
sometimes referred to as "good cholesterol". These balances are
mostly genetically determined, but can be changed by body build,
medications, food choices, and other factors.[47] Resistin, a protein
secreted by fat tissue, has been shown to increase the production of
LDL in human liver cells and also degrades LDL receptors in the
liver. As a result, the liver is less able to clear cholesterol from the
bloodstream. Resistin accelerates the accumulation of LDL in
arteries, increasing the risk of heart disease. Resistin also adversely
impacts the effects of statins, the main cholesterol-reducing drug
used in the treatment and prevention of cardiovascular disease.[48]

http://en.wikipedia.org/wiki/Cholesterol#Clinical_significance

CHRONIC
1.   (of an illness) Persisting for a long time or constantly

recurring
- ○ chronic bronchitis
2. (of a person) Having such an illness
- ○ a chronic asthmatic
3. (of a problem) Long-lasting and difficult to eradicate
- ○ the school suffers from chronic overcrowding
4. (of a person) Having a particular bad habit
- ○ a chronic liar

(Google Dictionary, 2012)

CO-MORBIDITIES
In medicine, comorbidity (literally "additional morbidity") is either the presence of one or more disorders (or diseases) in addition to a primary disease or disorder, or the effect of such additional disorders or diseases.

(http://en.wikipedia.org/wiki/Comorbidities)
Morbidity
The condition of being diseased, sick, [or injured]*.
(http://www.specialweb.com/aids/glossary.html)

In this book, the primary disease we are concerned with is obesity. The additional diseases can be any other chronic, active disease or permanent injury. This includes but is not limited to: diabetes, arthritis, fibromyalgia, depression, hepatitis, cardio-vascular disease, cancer, high blood pressure, paralysis, and a host of others. Please see your doctor before taking any diet, exercise, or mental health advice from anyone, including me.
*added by author

COGNITIVE DISSONANCE
The state of having inconsistent thoughts, beliefs, or attitudes, esp. as relating to behavioral decisions and attitude change.
• Cognitive dissonance is an uncomfortable feeling caused by holding conflicting ideas simultaneously. The theory of cognitive dissonance proposes that people have a motivational drive to reduce dissonance. They do this by changing their attitudes, beliefs, and actions. Festinger, L. (1957). ...
(http://en.wikipedia.org/wiki/Cognitive_dissonance)
(google dictionary, 2012)

COMPLETE BLOOD COUNTS (CBC)
A complete blood count (CBC), also known as full blood count (FBC) or full blood exam (FBE) or blood panel, is a test panel requested by a doctor or other medical professional that gives information about the cells in a patient's blood. A scientist or lab technician performs the requested testing and provides the requesting medical professional with the results of the CBC.

Alexander Vastem is widely regarded as being the first person to use the complete blood count for clinical purposes.[citation needed] Reference ranges used today stem from his clinical trials in the early 1960s.

The cells that circulate in the bloodstream are generally divided into three types: white blood cells (leukocytes), red blood cells (erythrocytes), and platelets (thrombocytes). Abnormally high or low counts may indicate the presence of many forms of disease, and hence blood counts are amongst the most commonly performed blood tests in medicine, as they can provide an overview of a patient's general health status. A CBC is routinely performed during annual physical examinations in some jurisdictions.

Many disease states are heralded by changes in the blood count:
- leukocytosis can be a sign of infection.
- thrombocytopenia can result from drug toxicity.
- pancytopenia is generally referred to as the result of decreased production from the bone   marrow, and is a common complication of cancer chemotherapy.

For a fairly complete list of CBC results within normal ranges see:
http://en.wikipedia.org/wiki/Reference_ranges_for_blood_tests#Hematology

http://en.wikipedia.org/wiki/Complete_blood_count#Results

COMPLEX OBESITY

Despite the fact that obesity is a complex disease, it is made much more so by the additional diseases we sometimes have. For example, diabetes or arthritis are diseases independent of obesity, but they make obesity much more difficult to manage. When you have both obesity and another independent disease, I have termed this Complex Obesity.

COMPULSIVITY

1.   Resulting from or relating to an irresistible urge, especially one that is against one's   conscious wishes
    ◦   compulsive eating
2.   (of a person) Acting as a result of such an urge
    ◦   a compulsive liar
(GoogleDictionary.com)

DIET

1.   The kinds of food that a person, animal, or community habitually eats
    ◦   a vegetarian diet
    ◦   a specialist in diet
2.   A special course of food to which one restricts oneself, either to lose weight or for medical reasons

◦ I'm going on a diet
3. (of food or drink) With reduced fat or sugar content
◦ diet soft drinks
4. A regular occupation or series of activities in which one participates
◦ a healthy diet of classical music
(Google Dictionary, 2012).

DIET GURU
A Guru is a recognized leader in some field or of some movement; "a guru of economics"
The term "guru" has been so overused in our culture that is has little to no real meaning.
A Diet Guru is a recognized leader in the diet or weight loss industry. Today there are many self-proclaimed diet gurus. No one has formally recognized them for their work in the field or study of obesity but they have taken the monicker for themselves in order to appear more credible.

DISORDERED EATING
"Disordered eating is a classification (within DSM-IV-TR, used in the health-care field) to describe a wide range of irregular eating behaviors that do not warrant a diagnosis of a specific eating disorder such as anorexia nervosa or bulimia nervosa. Affected people may be diagnosed with an eating disorder not otherwise specified. A change in eating patterns can also be caused by other mental disorders (e.g. clinical depression), or by factors that are generally considered to be unrelated to mental disorders (e.g. extreme homesickness).[1]
Some people consider disordered-eating patterns that are not the result of a specific eating disorder to be less serious than symptoms of disorders such as anorexia nervosa. Others note that individual cases may involve serious problems with food and body image. Additionally, certain types of disordered eating can include symptoms from both classic cases of anorexia and bulimia, making disordered eating just as dangerous.
Some counselors specialize in disordered-eating patterns. The recognition that some people have eating problems that do not fit into the scope of specific eating disorders makes it possible for a larger proportion of people who have eating problems to receive help.
Disordered eating affects the lives of up to 5 million adults and their families in the United States (Hewitt et al., 2001). Problematic

eating behaviour may emerge during childhood or adolescence and persist into mid and late-adulthood, or first emerge during mid-life. (Berry & Marcus, 2000; Chavez & Insel, 2007; Fairburn et al., 2003; Streigel-Moore & Bulik, 2007).[1] Disordered eating behaviors are associated with a number of harmful behavioral, physical, and psychological consequences, including poorer dietary quality, weight gain and obesity onset, depressive symptoms, and the onset of eating disorders. Thus, it is important to identify strategies for the prevention of disordered eating behaviors.[2]"
http://en.wikipedia.org/wiki/Disordered_eating

DR. KAHAN'S ARTICLE
If you would like to read Dr. Kahan's article, you can find it at the link provided below.
http://www.huffingtonpost.com/scott-kahan-md/obesity-disease_b_861087.html

DUMPING SYNDROME
This weight loss surgery side effect includes weakness, dizziness, flushing and warmth, nausea and palpitation immediately or shortly after eating and produced by abnormally rapid emptying of the stomach especially in individuals who have had part of the stomach removed.
Commonly referred to by these terms: Dump, Dumping.

EATING DISORDERS
Eating disorders refer to a group of conditions defined by abnormal eating habits that may involve either insufficient or excessive food intake to the detriment of an individual's physical and mental health. Bulimia nervosa, anorexia nervosa, and binge eating disorder are the most common specific forms in the United Kingdom [also true in the U.S.].

- Anorexia nervosa (AN), characterized by refusal to maintain a healthy body weight, an obsessive fear of gaining weight, and an unrealistic perception of current body weight. However, some patients can suffer from Anorexia nervosa unconsciously. These patients are classified under "atypical eating disorders". Anorexia can cause menstruation to stop, and often leads to bone loss, loss of skin integrity, etc. It greatly stresses the heart, increasing the risk of heart attacks and related heart problems. The risk of death is greatly increased in individuals with this disease.[15]

- Bulimia nervosa (BN), characterized by recurrent binge

eating followed by compensatory behaviors such as purging (self-induced vomiting, excessive use of laxatives/diuretics, or excessive exercise). Fasting and over exercise may also used as a method of purging following a binge.

- Binge eating disorder (BED) or 'compulsive overeating', characterized by binge eating, without compensatory behavior. This type of eating disorder is even more common than Bulimia or anorexia. This disorder does not have a category of people in which it can develop. In fact, this disorder can develop in a range of ages and is unbiased to classes.[16][17]

- Compulsive overeating, (COE) characteristic of binge eating disorder, in which people tend to eat more than necessary resulting in more stress. This is mainly caused by 'binge eating disorder'.[18]

- Purging disorder, characterized by recurrent purging to control weight or shape in the absence of binge eating episodes.

- Rumination, characterized by involving the repeated painless regurgitation of food following a meal which is then either re-chewed and re-swallowed, or discarded.

- Diabulimia, characterized by the deliberate manipulation of insulin levels by diabetics in an effort to control their weight.

- Food maintenance, characterized by a set of aberrant eating behaviors of children in foster care.[19]

- Eating disorders not otherwise specified (EDNOS) can refer to a number of disorders. It can refer to a female individual who suffers from anorexia but still has her period, someone who may be at a "healthy weight", but who has anorexic thought patterns and behaviors, it can mean the sufferer equally participates in some anorexic as well as bulimic behaviors (sometimes referred to as purge-type anorexia), or to any combination of eating disorder behaviors which do not directly put them in a separate category.

- Pica, characterized by a compulsive craving for eating, chewing or licking non-food items or foods containing no nutrition. These can include such things as chalk, paper, plaster, paint chips, baking soda, starch, glue, rust, ice, coffee grounds, and cigarette ashes. These individuals cannot distinguish a difference between food and non food items.

- Night eating syndrome, characterized by morning anorexia, evening polyphagia (abnormally increased appetite for consumption of food (frequently associated withinsomnia, and injury to the hypothalamus).

- Orthorexia nervosa, a term used by Steven Bratman to characterize an obsession with a "pure" diet, where it interferes with a person's life.

Several of the above mentioned disorders, such as diabulimia, food maintenance syndrome and orthorexia nervosa, are not currently recognized as mental disorders in any of the medical manuals, such as the ICD-10[20] or the DSM-IV.[21]
(http://en.wikipedia.org/wiki/Eating_disorder)

ENDORPHINS
A natural painkiller: a substance in the brain that attaches to the same cell receptors that morphine does. Endorphins are released when severe injury occurs, often abolishing all sensation of pain.
bing.com · Bing Dictionary

FOOD CHAIN
In ecology, the sequence of transfers of matter and energy from organism to organism in the form of food. Food chains intertwine locally into a food web because most organisms consume more than one type of animal or plant. Plants, which convert solar energy to food by photosynthesis, are the primary food source. In a predator chain, a plant-eating animal is eaten by a flesh-eating animal. In a parasite chain, a smaller organism consumes part of a larger host and may itself be parasitized by even smaller organisms. In a saprophytic chain, microorganisms live on dead organic matter.

Because energy, in the form of heat, is lost at each step, or trophic level, chains do not normally encompass more than four or five trophic levels.

People can increase the total food supply by cutting out one step in the food chain: instead of consuming animals that eat cereal grains, the people themselves consume the grains. Because the food chain is made shorter, the total amount of energy available to the final consumers is increased.
(http://www.britannica.com/EBchecked/topic/212636/food-chain)

HERE'S WHY SURGEONS DON'T REPLACE KNEES AT 40
This is why the surgeons I saw said that they would not replace my knees while I was in my 40s. Artificial knees, for the most part, last only about 10 years. Those knees wear out and the more active you are, the faster they wear out. If you are younger it is assumed that you are more active than an old person.

The reason this is important is that when they place an artificial knee into your body they have to tether it to the existing bones around the area. They can only do that a couple times before those surrounding bones falter. So, if you get the surgery in your 40s you are going to need as many as 5 or 6 replacements before you die. If you are younger, you will need them replaced even more often than every 10 years. You see where the problem comes in.

There is a bigger problem with artificial knee joints than that. An older person (someone 75+ years old) might benefit from knee replacement surgery because their expectations for movement are usually lower than a younger person's expectations. I wanted to run again! But the problem is that artificial knees are not appropriately built for running on. They are simply built to reduce pain and allow a person to be able to walk with less pain. That's far more appropriate for an older person than for someone in their 40s.

There are cases of people who have had knee replacement surgery at much younger ages. And I even know a woman who jogs on her artificial knees. It can be done. And I suspect as the technology improves it will become more and more the norm. But for now, it isn't the norm. It is the exception.

HIGH FRUCTOSE CORN SYRUP (HFCS)
A sweetener made by processing corn syrup to increase the level of fructose, usually to between 42% and 55% of the total sugar, with the balance being glucose. It is used extensively as a sweetener in processed foods and soft drinks, particularly soda and baked goods, but it is included also in many foods not normally thought of as sweet foods.
(http://medical-dictionary.thefreedictionary.com/high-fructose+corn+syrup)

HIGH TRIGLYCERIDES
Triglycerides are a type of fat found in your blood. Your body uses them for energy.

You need some triglycerides for good health. But high triglycerides can raise your risk of heart disease and may be a sign of metabolic syndrome.

Metabolic syndrome is the combination of high blood pressure, high blood sugar, too much fat around the waist, low HDL ("good") cholesterol, and high triglycerides. Metabolic syndrome increases your risk for heart disease, diabetes, and stroke.

A blood test that measures your cholesterol also measures your triglycerides. For a general idea about your triglycerides level, compare your test results to the following:
- Normal is less than 150.

- Borderline-high is 150 to 199.
- High is 200 to 499.
- Very high is 500 or higher.

What causes high triglycerides?

High triglycerides are usually caused by other conditions, such as:

- Obesity.
- Poorly controlled diabetes.
- An under active thyroid (hypothyroidism).
- Kidney disease.
- Regularly eating more calories than you burn.
- Drinking a lot of alcohol.

Certain medicines may also raise triglycerides. These medicines include:

- Tamoxifen.
- Steroids.
- Beta-blockers.
- Diuretics.
- Estrogen.
- Birth control pills.

In a few cases, high triglycerides also can run in families.

What are the symptoms?

High triglycerides usually don't cause symptoms.

But if your high triglycerides are caused by a genetic condition, you may see fatty deposits under your skin. These are called xanthomas (say "zan-THOH-muhs").

How can you lower your high triglycerides?

You can make diet and lifestyle changes to help lower your levels.

- Stay at a healthy weight.
- Limit fats and sugars in your diet.
- Be more active.
- Quit smoking.
- Limit alcohol.

You also may need medicine to help lower your triglycerides, but your doctor likely will ask you to try diet and lifestyle changes first.

http://www.webmd.com/cholesterol-management/tc/high-triglycerides-overview

HOMEOSTASIS

1.   (physiology) The ability of a system or living organism to adjust its internal environment to maintain a stable equilibrium;

such as the ability of warm-blooded animals to maintain a constant temperature.
2.   Such a dynamic equilibrium or balance.
(http://en.wiktionary.org/wiki/homeostasis)

INFLAMMATION
"Inflammation in the body is a normal and healthy response to injury or attack by germs. We can see it, feel it and measure it as local heat, redness, swelling, and pain. This is the body's way of getting more nourishment and more immune activity into an area that needs to fend off infection or heal. But inflammation isn't always helpful. It also has great destructive potential, which we see when the immune system mistakenly targets the body's own tissues in (autoimmune) diseases like type 1 diabetes, rheumatoid arthritis and lupus.
Whole-body inflammation refers to chronic, imperceptible, low-level inflammation. Mounting evidence suggests that over time this kind of inflammation sets the foundation for many serious, age-related diseases including heart disease, cancer and neurodegenerative conditions such as Alzheimer's and Parkinson's diseases. Recent evidence indicates that whole-body inflammation may also contribute to psychological disorders, especially depression.
The extent of this chronic inflammation is influenced by genetics, a sedentary lifestyle, too much stress, and exposure to environmental toxins such as secondhand tobacco smoke. Diet has a huge impact, so much so that I believe that most people in our part of the world go through life in a pro-inflammatory state as a result of what they eat. I'm convinced that the single most important thing you can do to counter chronic inflammation is to stop eating refined, processed and manufactured foods."
from   http://www.drweil.com/drw/u/QAA401013/Reducing-Whole-Body-Inflammation.html

INFLAMMATION MARKERS
C-reactive protein (CRP) is a protein found in the blood, the levels of which rise in response to inflammation (i.e. C-reactive protein is an acute-phase protein). Its physiological role is to bind to phosphocholine expressed on the surface of dead or dying cells (and some types of bacteria) in order to activate the complement system via the C1Q complex.[1]
CRP is synthesized by the liver[2] in response to factors released by macrophages and fat cells (adipocytes).[3] It is a member of the

pentraxin family of proteins.[2] It is not related to C-peptide or protein C. C-reactive protein was the first pattern recognition receptor (PRR) to be identified.[4]

CRP is used mainly as a marker of inflammation. Apart from liver failure, there are few known factors that interfere with CRP production.[2]

Measuring and charting CRP values can prove useful in determining disease progress or the effectiveness of treatments. Blood, usually collected in a serum-separating tube, is analysed in a medical laboratory or at the point of care. Various analytical methods are available for CRP determination, such as ELISA, immunoturbidimetry, rapid immunodiffusion, and visual agglutination.

A high-sensitivity CRP (hs-CRP) test measures low levels of CRP using laser nephelometry. The test gives results in 25 minutes with a sensitivity down to 0.04 mg/L.

Normal concentration in healthy human serum is usually lower than 10 mg/L, slightly increasing with aging. Higher levels are found in late pregnant women, mild inflammation and viral infections (10–40 mg/L), active inflammation, bacterial infection (40–200 mg/L), severe bacterial infections and burns (>200 mg/L).[23]

CRP is a more sensitive and accurate reflection of the acute phase response than the ESR (Erythrocyte Sedimentation Rate). The half-life of CRP is constant. Therefore, CRP level is mainly determined by the rate of production (and hence the severity of the precipitating cause). In the first 24 h, ESR may be normal and CRP elevated. CRP returns to normal more quickly than ESR in response to therapy.

http://en.wikipedia.org/wiki/C-reactive_protein

IRS LAW ON OBESITY

Internal Revenue Service: (IRS) the bureau of the United States Treasury Department responsible for tax collections.

Rev. Rul. 2002–19, page 778.

Medical expenses. Uncompensated amounts paid by individuals for participation in a weight-loss program as treatment for a specific disease or diseases (including obesity) diagnosed by a physician are expenses for medical care under section 213 of the Code. The cost of purchasing diet food items is not deductible under section 213. Rev. Ruls. 55–261 and 79–151 distinguished.

INVESTIGATOR SPONSORED RESEARCH COMPANY

What these companies do in many cases can contrast with scientifically based, peer-reviewed, or academic research. There are companies whose sole purpose is to support the claims of businesses about their products or services.

Businesses pay companies to research their products, which is a direct conflict of interest. Investigator-Sponsored Research can be legitimate. This is another area that can be difficult for a lay person to decipher. My rule of thumb is that conflicts or potential conflicts of interests must be made obvious by the researcher and by the publisher of that research. If the researcher gains from their work, it must be disclosed. This is common practice required for academic research.

ISOMETRIC EXERCISES

"Isometric exercise or isometrics are a type of strength training in which the joint angle and muscle length do not change during contraction (compared to concentric or eccentric contractions, called dynamic/isotonic movements). Isometrics are done in static positions, rather than being dynamic through a range of motion. Isometric exercise is a form of exercise involving the static contraction of a muscle without any visible movement in the angle of the joint. This is reflected in the name; the term "isometric" combines Greek the prefixes "iso" (same) with "metric" (distance), meaning that in these exercises the length of the muscle and the angle of the joint do not change, though contraction strength may be varied.[1] This is in contrast to isotonic contractions, in which the contraction strength does not change, though the muscle length and joint angle do."

http://en.wikipedia.org/wiki/Isometric_exercise

KALE

Boasting an incredible 206% of the recommended amount of Vitamin A, this green leafy veggie is amazingly versatile. It's also high in Calcium (9% of recommended daily intake) and has 6% of your daily Iron. With 134% of Vitamin C kale has a lot to offer! Besides that it is crunchy, works well with almost any flavor you want to add to it, and can be eaten cooked or raw. It has a very low glycemic index rating too (It's a 3 our of 100)!

(http://nutritiondata.self.com/)

MAIN EFFECTS

This is a term I borrowed from the research world and applied it to refer to the intended consequences of a treatment. For example, weight loss is the intended effect or main effect of weight loss surgery. As opposed to the side effects which include dumping syndrome and dehydration, hair loss, indigestion and the list goes on.

METOMORPHISIS

The process of changing from one form to another; e.g., in insects, from the larval stage to the pupal stage to the reproductive adult stage.

http://www2.estrellamountain.edu/faculty/farabee/biobk/BioBoo kglossM.html

MORBID OBESITY

Obesity is generally thought of in classifications. Class I Obesity is severe obesity. Class II is Morbid Obesity, Class III is Super Obesity.

BMI	Classification
< 18.5	underweight
18.5–24.9	normal weight
25.0–29.9	overweight
30.0–34.9	class I obesity
35.0–39.9	class II obesity
≥ 40.0	class III obesity

http://en.wikipedia.org/wiki/Obesity

MONOSODIUM GLUTAMATE (MSG)

The following is a quote from Livestrong.com. "The trade name of monosodium glutamate, according to California State University at Dominguez Hills, is sodium hydrogen glutamate. Because MSG is the sodium salt of the amino acid glutamic acid, whenever glutamic acid is listed on a food label, the food always contains MSG, according to Vanderbilt University. MSG may also be listed as monopotassium glutamate or simply as glutamate.

Food that lists the ingredient yeast extract always contains MSG, according to Vanderbilt University. Although MSG may also be labeled autolyzed yeast, yeast food or yeast nutrient, the common name including the word yeast currently used in processed foods to avoid listing the ingredient as monosodium glutamate is yeast extract. Avoid foods with yeast extract if you have adverse reactions to MSG, even though you find the enhanced flavor highly appealing.

Hydrolyzed protein is a common term used for MSG, whether it is hydrolyzed vegetable protein, animal protein or plant protein, according to the department of nutrition and exercise science at Bastyr University. Vanderbilt University adds that any food ingredient listed as hydrolyzed, protein-fortified, ultra-pasteurized, fermented or enzyme-modified is often MSG, or creates free glutamic acid during processing. These other names include soy protein isolate, soy protein concentrate, whey protein, whey protein concentrate, whey protein isolate, autolyzed plant protein, hydrolyzed oat flour and textured protein. With so many names for MSG, if you are sensitive or allergic to MSG, make a list of these alternative names and consult it when you go shopping."

Read more: http://www.livestrong.com/article/377482-other-names-for-msg-or-monosodium-glutamate/#ixzz234nCsm00

NEW YORK STATE DEPARTMENT OF HEATLH

http://www.health.ny.gov/

http://www.health.ny.gov/prevention/obesity/

NIGHTSHADE VEGETABLES

Nightshades include fruits and vegetables that contain alkaloids and many in their immature states are toxic and even poisonous. Many nightshades are poisonous and in large doses fatal to horses and cows. Examples of edible nightshade vegetables are potatoes, eggplant, bell pepper, Italian pepper, chile pepper, tomato and tomatillo. Some fruits are considered nightshades including gooseberry, the goji berry, and pepino.

Nightshade plants are linked to increases in arthritis pain and many people with arthritis avoid eating them.

Read more: List of Nightshade Vegetables & Fruits | eHow.com http://www.ehow.com/info_7841462_list-nightshade-vegetables-fruits.html#ixzz2IcikDYY0

OBESE

A BMI greater than 30 kg/m2 (Okoro, Sintler, & Khan, 2009).

BMI	Classification
< 18.5	underweight
18.5–24.9	normal weight
25.0–29.9	overweight
30.0–34.9	class I obesity
35.0–39.9	class II obesity
≥ 40.0	class III obesity

OVERWEIGHT
A BMI greater than 25 kg/m2 (Okoro, Sintler, & Khan, 2009).

BMI	Classification
< 18.5	underweight
18.5–24.9	normal weight
25.0–29.9	overweight
30.0–34.9	class I obesity
35.0–39.9	class II obesity
≥ 40.0	class III obesity

PHYTOCHEMICALS
Chemical compounds that occur naturally in plants (phyto means "plant" in Greek), are responsible for color and organoleptic properties, such as the deep purple of blueberries and smell of garlic. The term is generally used to refer to those chemicals that may have biological significance but are not established as essential nutrients.[1] Scientists estimate that there may be as many as 10,000 different phytochemicals having the potential to affect diseases such as cancer, stroke or metabolic syndrome.
http://en.wikipedia.org/wiki/Phytochemical

PRINCETON RESEARCH OF SWEETENERS
"A Princeton University research team has demonstrated that all sweeteners are not equal when it comes to weight gain: Rats with access to high-fructose corn syrup gained significantly more weight than those with access to table sugar, even when their overall caloric intake was the same.

In addition to causing significant weight gain in lab animals, long-term consumption of high-fructose corn syrup also led to abnormal increases in body fat, especially in the abdomen, and a rise in circulating blood fats called triglycerides. The researchers say the work sheds light on the factors contributing to obesity trends in the United States.

"Some people have claimed that high-fructose corn syrup is no different than other sweeteners when it comes to weight gain and obesity, but our results make it clear that this just isn't true, at least under the conditions of our tests," said psychology professor Bart Hoebel, who specializes in the neuroscience of appetite, weight and sugar addiction. "When rats are drinking high-fructose corn syrup at levels well below those in soda pop, they're becoming obese -- every single one, across the board. Even when rats are fed a high-fat diet, you don't see this; they don't all gain extra weight.'"

from
http://www.princeton.edu/main/news/archive/S26/91/22K07/

click the link read the entire story.

REACTIVE HYPOGLYCEMIA

Reactive hypoglycemia, or postprandial hypoglycemia, is a medical term describing recurrent episodes of symptomatic hypoglycemia occurring within 4 hours after a high carbohydrate meal (or oral glucose load) in people who do not have diabetes. It is thought to represent a consequence of excessive insulin release triggered by the carbohydrate meal but continuing past the digestion and disposal of the glucose derived from the meal.

Symptoms vary according to individuals' hydration level and sensitivity to the rate and/or magnitude of decline of their blood glucose concentration. Some of the food-induced hypoglycemia symptoms include:
- Double vision or blurry vision
- Unclear thinking
- Sleeping Trouble
- heart palpitation or fibrillation
- fatigue
- dizziness
- light-headedness
- sweating
- headaches
- depression
- nervousness

- irritability
- tremors
- flushing
- craving sweets
- increased appetite
- nausea, vomiting
- panic attack
- numbness/coldness in the extremities
- confusion
- coma can be a result in severe untreated episodes

(http://en.wikipedia.org/wiki/Reactive_hypoglycemia)

RESTING PULSE RATES

The resting heart rate (HRrest) is measured while the subject is at rest but awake, and not having recently exerted himself or herself. The typical resting heart rate in adults is 60–80 beats per minute (bpm).[2] Resting heart rates below 60 bpm may be referred to as bradycardia, while rates above 100 bpm at rest may be called tachycardia.

Fitness training can lead to cardiovascular changes including hypertrophy of the left ventricle and angiogenesis within muscle tissue. This leads to a state known as athletic heart syndrome, as distinct from the pathological enlargements of the ventricles in ventricular hypertrophy. Resting heart rates for athletes can be well below 60, with values of below 40 bpm not unheard of. The cyclist Miguel Indurain had a resting heart rate of 28 bpm.[3]

Average resting heart rate is correlated with age:[4]

http://en.wikipedia.org/wiki/Heart_rate#Resting_heart_rate

REVISION SURGERY

Revision Weight Loss Surgery is a surgical procedure that is performed on patients who have already undergone a form of bariatric surgery, and have either had complications from such surgery or have not successfully achieved significant weight loss results from the initial surgery.[1] Procedures are usually performed laparoscopically, though open surgery may be required if prior bariatric surgery has resulted in extensive scarring.

With the increase in the number of weight loss surgeries performed every year,[2] there are growing numbers of individuals who have experienced an unsatisfactory result from their bariatric procedures.

StomaphyX revision is a completely endoscopic revision technique[12] used to tighten a stretched gastric pouch using internal sutures or fasteners. It may be used in patients who have had prior roux-en-Y gastric bypass surgery and have a stretched stomach pouch.

(http://en.wikipedia.org/wiki/Revision_weight_loss_surgery)

RHEUMATOID ARTHRITIS

rheu·ma·toid ar·thri·tis

A chronic progressive disease causing inflammation in the joints and resulting in painful deformity and immobility, esp. in the fingers, wrists, feet, and ankles

(Google Dictionary, 2012)

Various Web Definitions

• a chronic autoimmune disease with inflammation of the joints and marked deformities; something (possibly a virus) triggers an attack on the synovium by the immune system, which releases cytokines that stimulate an inflammatory reaction that can lead to the destruction of all components of the joint

http://wordnetweb.princeton.edu/perl/webwn?s=rheumatoid

• Rheumatoid Arthritis (RA) is a chronic, systemic inflammatory disorder that may affect many tissues and organs, but principally attacks synovial joints. ...

http://en.wikipedia.org/wiki/Rheumatoid_arthritis

• Disorder that is believed to result from an "autoimmune" process in which the body's immune system attacks itself. It is a system-wide disease that usually last for many years. In some patients, RA affects such organs as the heart, lungs, and eyes. Patients with active RA often feel feverish or ill.

http://www.pennmedicine.org/health_info/arthritis/000075.html

A crippling form of arthritis that begins with inflammation and thickening of the synovial membrane, followed by bone degeneration and disfigurement.

http://www.emc.maricopa.edu/faculty/farabee/biobk/biobookglossr.html

SIDE EFFECTS

In medicine, a side effect is an effect, whether therapeutic or adverse, that is secondary to the one intended; although the term is

predominantly employed to describe adverse effects, it can also apply to beneficial, but unintended...
(http://en.wikipedia.org/wiki/Side_effects)

SIMPLE OBESITY

This is a term I use for folks who suffer from the disease of obesity but do not have a co-existing disease. For example, there are a lot of folks out there who have obesity but not high blood pressure, or diabetes or any other obesity related disease. Neither do they endure an unrelated disease that impacts their ability to manage obesity. For example, I have Rheumatoid Arthritis. It is unrelated to obesity but makes obesity difficult to manage because it restricts my ability to exercise. There is nothing simple about obesity. All on its own it is a complex disease.

SUPER (OR MORBID) OBESITY

A body mass index (BMI) greater than 40 kg/m2 (Okoro, Sintler, & Khan, 2009).

TESTIMONIALS

In promotion and advertising, a testimonial consists of a written or spoken statement, sometimes from a public figure, sometimes from a private citizen, extolling the virtue of some product.

The FTC (Federal Trade Commission) in fact found that in US businesses an alarming number of testimonials were so fictitious and misleading that in Dec of 2009 they introduced a new set of rules governing testimonials.
http://en.wikipedia.org/wiki/Testimonial

THYROID COUNTS

Thyroid blood tests generally include determination of the levels of circulating thyroid hormones (Free T4 and Free T3 and thyroid stimulating hormone TSH). These tests, especially the TSH, are highly sensitive and reliable, and the levels of thyroid hormones or TSH do not fluctuate widely during the day, or from day to day. Hence it is highly unlikely that a significant disturbance of thyroid function (hypo or hyperthyroidism) is present if the TSH is normal, even if only a single TSH determination is carried out. The results of thyroid blood tests can be affected by other medications a patient may be taking, so be sure that this information is provided to your physician. Patients who are being treated for hyperthyroidism usually require more than just a TSH determination to assess their thyroid status, since the TSH level can remain low for a prolonged period of time, even as the hyperthyroidism is getting better and the levels of Free T4 and T3 are dropping.

to read more on the topic:
http://www.mythyroid.com/bloodtests.html

TRANS FATS

Trans fat is the common name for unsaturated fat with trans-isomer (E-isomer) fatty acid(s). Because the term refers to the configuration of a double carbon-carbon bond, trans fats are sometimes monounsaturated or polyunsaturated, but never saturated. Trans fats do exist in nature but also occur during the processing of polyunsaturated fatty acids in food production.[1]

The consumption of trans fats increases the risk of coronary heart disease[2][3] by raising levels of LDL cholesterol and lowering levels of "good" HDL cholesterol.[4] There is an ongoing debate about a possible differentiation between trans fats of natural origin and trans fats of vegetable origin but so far no scientific consensus was found. Two Canadian studies, that received funding by the Alberta Livestock and Meat Agency [5] and the Dairy Farmers of Canada,[6] have shown that the natural trans fat vaccenic acid, found in beef and dairy products, may have an opposite health effect and could actually be beneficial compared to hydrogenated vegetable shortening, or a mixture of pork lard and soy fat,[6] e.g. lowering total and LDL cholesterol and triglyceride levels.[7][8][9] In lack of recognized evidence and scientific agreement, nutritional authorities consider all trans fats as equally harmful for health [10] [11] [12] and recommend that consumption of trans fats be reduced to trace amounts.[13] [14]

(http://en.wikipedia.org/wiki/Transfat)

VEGAN

Being a vegan is the practice of abstaining from the use of animal products, particularly in diet, as well as an associated philosophy that rejects the commodity status of sentient animals. A follower of veganism is known as a vegan.

Distinctions are sometimes made between different types of vegans and veganism. A dietary vegan (or strict vegetarian) is one who eliminates animal products (not only meat and fish, but also dairy products, eggs and often honey, as well as other animal-derived substances) from their diet. The term ethical vegan or lifestyle vegan is often applied to someone who not only follows a vegan diet, but extends the vegan philosophy into other areas of their life. Another term used is environmental veganism, which refers to the rejection of animal products on the premise that the industrial exploitation of animals is environmentally damaging and unsustainable.

(http://en.wikipedia.org/wiki/Vegan)

WHITE KNUCKLING IT

Showing, experiencing, or causing very strong feelings of fear, anxiety, etc.

▪ a white-knuckle ride on a roller coaster ▪ I'm a white-knuckle flier/traveler. [=flying/traveling is very stressful for me] ▪ They rode their motorcycles at white-knuckle speeds.

http://www.merriam-webster.com/dictionary/white-knuckle

WORD OF MOUTH MARKETING

Word of Mouth Marketing (WOMM) refers to the marketing that can be gained by actively engaging customers to share insights with each other (create buzz that goes viral). WOMM has clearly been around since the inception of marketing, but has gained more prominence with the evolution of the internet, and the ease with which customers can share their stories. Web 2.0 technologies such as Blogs and News Readers are enabling WOMM. Discussion Boards have helped customers form communities. Good WOMM relies on great products that customers willingly evangelize. Marketers have been prone to try to 'effect' this by incentivizing 'fake' customers to talk about their products. This can backfire.

http://www.udel.edu/alex/dictionary.html

ABOUT THE AUTHOR

Carrie Hickman is married and is the mother of three sons and one little dog. She's working on her doctorate in Research Psychology while she writes books from her cabin in the woods just outside Seattle, Washington.